Special praise for the
A Day with

"With the dramatic increase in prescription opioid abuse, managing pain and addiction—particularly for people in recovery—has become a major medical issue in our society. Mel Pohl is addiction medicine's leader in this complex area. He has provided guidelines that improve clinical outcomes and decrease consequences for these multi-problem patients. His book will be valuable reading for all in our field who deal with the complex issue of pain and addiction."

David E. Smith, MD
Founder of Haight-Ashbury Free Medical Clinics of San Francisco
Past President of American Society of Addiction Medicine
Chief of Addiction Medicine Newport Academy
Author of Unchain Your Brain

· ·

Suffering is optional!

A Day without Pain offers this timely message to those with chronic pain (and their physicians). Dr. Pohl illuminates the approach to the chronic pain patient and shows us the medical, psychological, and chemical dependency issues that must be addressed in these individuals.

"Dr. Pohl's humane understanding of complex patients is well-described, with particular attention to the medical, neurochemical, psychodynamic, and spiritual modalities that bring recovery to these suffering patients. The emphasis on narcotic-free living is paramount.

"As a practitioner on the 'firing line' treating chronic pain patients, I heartily recommend *A Day without Pain* to anyone suffering with this mysterious illness, as well as their caregivers, family, and friends."

Herbert Malinoff, MD, FACP, FASAM
Back and Pain Center
Department of Anesthesiology
University of Michigan Medical Center
Ann Arbor, Michigan

Praise for the first edition of
A Day without Pain

"*A Day without Pain* is based on the principle of 'physician heal thyself.'

"Dr. Pohl 'walks the walk' and 'talks the talk' of a drug-free approach to chronic pain management. This refreshing approach to a huge problem is long overdue and will benefit thousands of patients who suffer from chronic pain."

Harry L. Haroutunian, MD
Physician Director, Residential Treatment
Licensed Professional Program and Clinical Diagnostic Evaluations
Betty Ford Center, Rancho Mirage, California

•••

"In *A Day without Pain*, Mel Pohl explores the experience of chronic pain—from its complex multi-faceted causes to its often devastating effect on lives. Most importantly, through the stories of his patients, he illustrates routes to recovering from chronic pain's disabling impact. Dr. Pohl's compassionate, holistic, grounded, and honest approach to treating pain and its emotional and behavioral consequences shines through this book. I highly recommend *A Day without Pain* for anyone suffering from chronic pain or watching a loved one suffer."

Jodie A. Trafton, Ph.D.
Research Health Science Specialist
VA Palo Alto Center for Health Care Evaluation
Assistant Clinical Professor (affiliated), Stanford University
Department of Psychiatry and Behavioral Sciences

•••

"If you or a loved one suffers from chronic pain or chronic pain syndrome, please read this wonderful book. Dr. Mel Pohl combines all of the helpful elements—a very personal investment, a research perspective, and that of a compassionate healer. As someone diagnosed with rheumatoid arthritis, I can only wish that Dr. Pohl had years ago been available to me as a teacher and a physician."

Cardwell C. Nuckols, MA, Ph.D.
Internationally recognized expert in behavioral medicine and addictions treatment
Longwood, Florida
Author of Healing an Angry Heart

A DAY
Without
PAIN

(REVISED AND UPDATED)

Mel Pohl, MD, FASAM

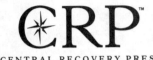

CENTRAL RECOVERY PRESS

CENTRAL RECOVERY PRESS

Central Recovery Press (CRP) is committed to publishing exceptional materials addressing addiction treatment, recovery, and behavioral health care, including original and quality books, audio/visual communications, and web-based new media. Through a diverse selection of titles, we seek to contribute a broad range of unique resources for professionals, recovering individuals and their families, and the general public.

For more information, visit www.centralrecoverypress.com.

Central Recovery Press, Las Vegas, NV
© 2008, 2011 by Central Recovery Press

Printed in the United States of America

17 16 15 14 13 12 11   1 2 3 4 5

ISBN-13: 978-1-936290-62-8 (paper)
ISBN-10: 1-936290-62-6

Publisher: Central Recovery Press
             3321 N Buffalo Drive
             Las Vegas, NV 89129

Images on pages: 46, 135, 136, 139, 140, 141, 143, 145, 148, 151, 160, 163, 177 ©2011 Jupiterimages Corporation. Used by permission. Image used on page 32 courtesy of NIDA. Image used on page 47 courtesy of Foundation for Recovery.

Cover design and interior by Sara Streifel, Think Creative Design

I dedicate this book to all of my best teachers—
the clients at Las Vegas Recovery Center—
for their courage and dedication to getting better.

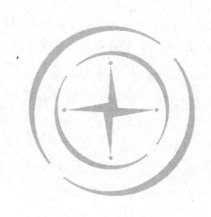

TABLE OF CONTENTS

To help you better understand some of the terminology in this book, a glossary has been included at the back for your reference. Words that are included in the glossary are bolded in the text.

A Day without Pain is an empowering book for people who thought that their lives could never be okay and they were destined to suffer. For the past two years I have had the benefit of consulting at Las Vegas Recovery Center, where Dr. Mel Pohl is the medical director and practicing physician. Clients arrive from all over the United States, usually having already experienced multiple methods of treatment. Most of the treatments have involved multiple surgeries, extensive dosing of pain medications, or some form of physical therapy. Sadly, these clients have not experienced relief from their situation and are often in worse condition. They have less mobility, more pain, and more depression, and some have developed addiction to painkillers. They arrive scared and angry, but anxiously hopeful—one more time—that someone can take their pain away, only to become more scared and angry when they are informed it isn't the pain that will be attended to, but the suffering.

It is the suffering that Dr. Pohl recognizes as the predominant focus for pain recovery. Recognizing that 80 percent of the pain experienced is emotional, the client is confronted with the reality that chronic pain doesn't go away. That is, in fact, what distinguishes it from acute pain. It is like an alarm clock that goes off and is stuck in a never-ending buzz mode, and it is the emotional responses over time that perpetuate the pain. No doubt this person has much to be emotional about; there is tremendous loss for him or her, and there is valid reason to feel anger, fear, sadness, loneliness, and so on. The paradox is that staying with the emotional pain, however righteous it is, perpetuates the physical pain.

It is clear to anyone who sees Dr. Pohl in his practice that his work requires a great amount of confidence in the knowledge of chronic pain and a great amount of empathy for the confused state of the person in pain. Those qualities are demonstrated in this book as he shares with you the conditions and complexities of chronic pain. The kindness and authority that Dr. Pohl exudes are also a major source of strength for helping professionals who must work with people when they are scared and engaging in self-destructive thinking and behaviors. This synergistic combination of helping traits is what assists the client in finding the willingness and the strength to let go of his or her crutches, both literal and metaphorical.

In *A Day without Pain* you will learn about the science of pain. Learning how chronic pain is different from acute pain is extremely validating for the person in pain. To see their lives portrayed via the stories of others with similar conditions, though the causes may vary, lessens the emotional isolation of those who have become totally self-absorbed. Understanding how the natural response of not wanting to move through the pain exacerbates the pain begins to make sense. But more importantly, being introduced to tools such as breathing, relaxation techniques, imagery, and movement offer not just hope but the beginning of distraction from the pain, a moment of relief. *A Day without Pain* describes in detail many valuable methods that work with chronic pain, encompassing approaches that address physical, psychological, and spiritual recovery.

Dr. Pohl speaks eloquently from a scientific viewpoint, but he writes in a style that is understandable to the lay reader. He addresses the benefits of using medications and the possible consequences of long-term use that complicate chronic pain. As an addiction specialist, he is experienced in recognizing when **tolerance**—a term used when more of the medication is needed to have the same effect as it did when the individual first used it—fuels addiction. He describes opioid-induced hyperalgesia, wherein a person feels more pain as a consequence of the opioids in his or her nervous system. This is "light bulb" information to the person who has been relying on medication to relieve the pain only to discover it is exacerbating his or her condition.

Everyone needs to be honored and respected for who they are as individuals, and by discussing the differences among gender influences, cultural influences, and the influence of family, the reader garners a comprehensive picture of how and why people respond differently to their physical states.

Family members struggle with maintaining their own autonomy, supporting their loved one in his or her independence, and yet their behavior often does the opposite of what is healthy for them or the loved one. The reader will discover how families are hardwired for their solicitous responses that only enable the person in pain to avoid taking more responsibility for his or her condition and, ultimately, his or her life. The dysfunction that is characteristic of addicted families is very common to families impacted by chronic pain—the person in pain becomes the central organizing feature around which all others revolve. Family members suffer their own losses. Communication and boundaries become distorted and blurred. Roles shift, and emotional and social isolation are a part of the changing system. Whether or not addiction has occurred in the family, the parallel paths offer a direction for healing the family system.

By being an active participant in your own recovery, embracing the knowledge that addressing the emotional nature of your suffering is the way out, and taking responsibility for your own actions with respect to functioning and medication use, you can well see that there need not be any victims.

Having seen it with my own eyes, I understand the passion that Dr. Pohl experiences when he sees clients who have lived for years in psychologically and physically demoralizing states recapture their autonomy. Neither they nor their families need any longer be hostage to their pain.

Claudia Black, Ph.D.
Addiction Specialist, Author of
It Will Never Happen to Me

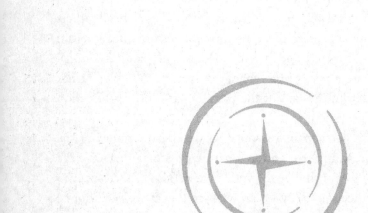

PREFACE TO THE REVISED EDITION

*"If I were to choose between pain and nothing,
I would choose pain."*

William Faulkner

In the three years since the first edition of this book was written, I have learned a lot about chronic pain through my work with Las Vegas Recovery Center's (LVRC) Pain Recovery Program, through my own personal experience with pain, and by studying research and available literature on this topic.

My pain has evolved as my body has aged. My back condition is a bit worse overall, with daily aches and pains that, in the old days, would have kept me in bed for a day or two, prompting a case of the "poor me's" as I looked for attention and sympathy. But my pain is not the only thing to have evolved. Fortunately, my response to pain has also evolved.

As a result, I have learned to work with those impulses to whine and complain or to look for attention and sympathy or to become scared and tighten up in an attempt to avoid the discomfort. Eventually, when I become more aware of what I am doing, I take a deep breath. Breath is the vehicle for slowing me down, focusing my attention on my body, thoughts, and emotions. Perhaps I'll simply stretch or do a three-minute meditation away from my daily routine. Usually it also entails an attitude adjustment: "Yes, it hurts, but I'm walking and functioning and went to the gym today." A simple shift of my focus from "me-centered" to "anything-other-than-me-centered" (could be you, could be the world, could be nature, could be music, could be God) distracts me from myself long enough to get me moving again. Today, I rarely find it fulfilling to wallow in self-pity or stay tightened up in a futile attempt to control something over which I am powerless.

An example of how I cope with pain happened recently when I went kayaking while on vacation in the Northwest. I felt like I was off on a three-hour tour to Gilligan's Island without a motor, a fantastic adventure. It started out gloriously—the promise of whales, dolphins, fellowship, and exquisite scenery. It actually ended up as three hours of fun and excitement, but the last two hours consisted of back-wrenching stroking in my two-man kayak. The last hour was miserable. I could feel the strain in my shoulders and back muscles as the relentless, yet necessary, stroking continued. And we still had a mile to go! I noticed my mind and what it created for me: stories of pulling a muscle and being out for the rest of the trip; a sense of helpless inadequacy because I was not younger and in better shape; and fear that my back was getting worse and soon I would not be able to participate in such activities, which for the most part are extremely enjoyable (except for that last mile!). The bottom line is that I was able to utilize the tools I have learned and taught folks over the years to settle my mind, focus on my breath in synchronicity with the stroking, tell my partner I had to rest periodically, and not beat myself up for being a "wuss."

Of course, we made it back alive, and I was sore for the next few days, but nothing incapacitating. I arranged to have a massage and made sure that my daily stretch lasted longer and involved the affected muscle groups. I used ice a few times, which was helpful in diminishing the discomfort. My approach to the use of medication is based on the concept of mindfulness: First, I notice the pain—without judgment, without extreme emotion, without creating a "story" about what it means—and always, I work with the breath. I usually put off taking anything for the pain in the moment. My instinct is to medicate with something like Tylenol or Advil, but with a few moments' delay and distraction by being involved in some activity, I usually *forget* the pain and don't need to medicate. I don't use opioids at all for my chronic pain, and my intention is to not do so.

One of the most common questions I am asked by clients and families in groups at Las Vegas Recovery Center is "What if I get hurt? What do I do about taking (or not taking) painkillers?" The instruction in *Pain Recovery: How to Find Balance and Reduce Suffering from Chronic Pain* (2009, Central Recovery Press) is to ask yourself three questions: "Do I *really* need to take opioids?" If the answer is yes, the next question is "Do I really, *really* need to take opioids?" And if the answer is yes, the next question is "Do I really, really, *really* need to take opioids?" If the answer to all three questions is yes, then call your sponsor, go to a meeting, and check your state of balance in the physical, emotional, mental, and spiritual areas of your life. If you decide to take medications on a short-term basis, then work out a plan to take as few as possible for as short a period as possible and have a trusted person hold the drugs.

My most noteworthy run-in with acute pain happened when I was in Lake Louise, Canada. I went there for a few days of R-and-R on my own. I went to an extraordinarily romantic spot called The Fairmont Chateau Lake Louise. I decided that being in Calgary at a conference merited a stay at the fabulous resort overlooking the lake, even though I was alone. If you've never been, I highly recommend it. There is a sparkling, crystalline, glacier-fed lake in the middle of steep mountains—a perfect setting to relax in and from which to explore the region.

I had just scheduled a hike, to be followed by an ATV (all-terrain vehicle) adventure at sunset, when I developed a pain in my right side that doubled me over. I became nauseated and threw up my breakfast. "Uh-oh," I thought, "what's going on?" I self-diagnosed appendicitis and called the concierge for information about medical help. It turned out the closest doctor was an hour's drive away. By that time I was hurting worse than I ever had before, so I decided to make the trip to Banff Community Hospital. Since I felt too sick to drive, I hired a local cab with a chatty driver who picked me up in a minivan. I persuaded the driver not to take the scenic route, although she insisted on stopping for the moose that was ambling up on the side of the road. "Aw, how cool. Look at him. We call him Harry and he comes to visit us."

I was in agony. "Cool. . . . OWWWW! Can we go now, please?"

When I got settled in the emergency room, the doctor examined me and suggested that I might actually have a kidney stone since I had blood in my urine. I refused his offer of morphine, because at that time the pain had subsided substantially (down to a five on a ten-point scale). In a few minutes, I was hit by a spasm that took my breath away. When I stopped retching, I answered yes to the three questions. I really, really, *really* needed medications. The pain by that time was a steady ten out of ten, definitely the worst pain I had ever experienced, incapacitating me to the point of feeling like I was going to pass out. Over the next thirty minutes, the doctor gave me three morphine injections and the pain subsided to a dull ache (three out of ten).

Eventually, I decided to return to my beautiful room alone on Lake Louise to spend my last night by the shimmering lake with my kidney stone. At 2:00 a.m., the pain recurred at an eight-of-ten level. I considered getting dressed and driving back to the emergency room, but I got by with Percocet 10 mg. I think I used six tablets and hardly slept that night. I called my sponsor, and it was fortunate for both of us that he was up at that hour. The next day I spoke with some recovery friends for support, prayed a lot, and survived to see the sun rise over the glacier. I was thrilled to observe the staggering beauty between spasms of pain.

The stone passed and kept me miserable for the better part of a week. (I am teased by friends relentlessly because it was only a few millimeters in size—tiny, but capable nonetheless of causing me significant misery.) As it passed, it left me exhausted, horribly constipated from the medications, and, I am grateful to say, with no desire to continue the opioids.

This is a case of acute pain being partially suppressed to a tolerable level by potent opioid medications, which continuously wore off and needed to be repeated for me to reenter a state of pain reduction. When the stone passed, the need for medications did, too. I noted a vague, fond memory of the mood-enhancing effect of the intravenous morphine, but had enough recovery in place to ensure that I did not "romance" the high or wish actively to repeat it. I was completely open about it, talking about my experience again and again with my twelve-step buddies, so much so that I was rewarded with some good laughs. And, mercifully, this episode of acute pain was over.

Those of us with chronic pain are not so lucky. The pain persists long after it serves any function. There's no stone causing obstruction that will eventually pass. The bulging disc in my back isn't notifying me of anything important like "If I move it, it is likely to cause worse damage," or "I need to protect myself." It's just there—annoyingly, persistently, aggravatingly there. At times I loathe it; other times I cry about it; but mostly, I accept it. It's just there.

I've updated this book because over the last three years I've learned much about chronic pain, and I believe the solutions I present in both editions work. I have come to embrace my pain, not as a friend or lover or enemy, but as a part of me. While my pain does not identify me, it *is* a part of me, and through my work, both as a practitioner and a person living with chronic pain, I know I would not be the person I am today without having gone through the experiences I have encountered. I hope you will find in these pages the solutions you have sought and learn how to live a day without pain.

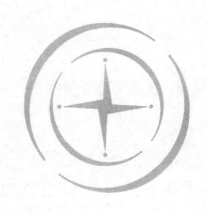

FOREWORD TO THE FIRST EDITION

A Day without Pain is a refreshing and comprehensive look at the issues impacting patients with chronic pain who have been searching for effective strategies to treat the many layers of this disease. On these pages there are tools outlined that have worked effectively in our practice for many years. We have a very strong emphasis not only on physical recovery and reduction of pain, but also on emotional, behavioral, and spiritual recovery.

I had been practicing addiction medicine for many years when my office began seeing patients referred by physicians who traditionally provide treatment for chronic pain. These colleagues were seeking help to detox their patients from the copious amount of medications they took to help fight their pain. Patients weren't improving despite escalating regimens of opioids and other drugs; pain levels were high, and functioning was suboptimal. Patient families were distressed and the physicians were at a loss. Patients were miserable. They often were angry, frustrated, mistrustful, scared, confused, and still in pain!

Despite evidence that pain medications were not working well, patients insisted on maintaining their use, repeatedly claiming, "If I didn't have pain, I wouldn't be taking them," or "My doctor prescribed them." And once the patients entered treatment for addiction, it got even worse. They felt misunderstood and mislabeled.

In our clinic, which consists of a small staff including a physician, pain psychologist, nurse practitioner, and social worker, we found that counseling staff, too, felt unprepared to respond to these patients. They asked, "Are these patients addicts? Are they in denial? What were the doctors thinking when prescribing all this medication? Should we even be looking at these medications? Don't the patients deserve to live pain-free?"

Our clinicians attempted to sort out addiction from other issues, referring pain problems right back to our medical staff. There seemed to be some type of sacred ground not to be trodden upon by nonmedical staff. They wanted "medical" to fix it. Unfortunately, medical staff was looking for help, too.

While we're not suggesting patients with chronic pain are addicts, it is important to note the similarities between the ramifications of chronic pain syndrome and the consequences of addiction. These similarities are outlined in Chapter Two of *A Day without Pain*. This chapter explains issues associated with living in chronic pain for longer than six months, which very often include depression, anger, worry, discouragement, irritability, sleep difficulties, financial problems, disturbed relationships, withdrawal from activities, inability to concentrate, memory deficits, sexual problems, diminished self-esteem, secondary physical problems, avoidance of work and leisure activities, and negative attitudes.

These consequences are very familiar to addiction counselors. No wonder health care providers need help. No wonder lives fall apart. No wonder relationships suffer or end. Something much, much bigger has taken control. In *A Day without Pain* it is called the "beast," or chronic pain syndrome.

In untold numbers of cases, patients suffering from chronic pain syndrome no longer obtain relief simply by taking pain medications. Dosages of medications are often increased to mind-boggling levels in the patient's search for relief.

Geri, a forty-six-year-old woman, at age twenty-five sustained three compression fractures of her back when she attempted suicide by jumping from five stories. She came to our clinic on a medication regimen that was no longer helpful. She was taking *four* prescribed opioids: Oxycontin (long-acting oxycodone), 80 milligrams, 6 tablets three times per day (which she chewed, looking for immediate relief); Norco (hydrocodone), 10/325, 4 tablets twice daily; Methadone, 40–60 milligrams daily; and Actiq (fentanyl) suckers, 1600 micrograms, 15–20 per day. She also was prescribed two sedatives/muscle relaxants: Valium (diazepam), 60–70 milligrams per day; and Soma (carisoprodol), 350 milligrams twice daily. She was unable to work due to the pain, as well as to the confusion and memory loss that were attributed to the side effects of the medications. Today she is on minimal medication and works as a job coach for physically and emotionally disabled clients, goes to school and church, volunteers, attends twelve-step meetings, and is involved in a softball league.

As so succinctly described in this book, in order to recover from the "beast," patients must become fully involved in their treatment. There are no passive patients in our pain clinic. Using many of the tools and techniques described in this book, we, too, have been successfully assisting patients obtain higher levels of functioning and quality of life by treating the *whole* patient and insisting upon full participation in treatment, including emotional and physical work. When chronic pain strikes, treatment must be aimed at biological, psychological, social, and spiritual aspects of the individual.

Specialists in chronic pain and the authors of *A Day without Pain* understand that chronic pain is a disease process that stands alone. Knowledgeable and compassionate providers must accurately diagnose and treat addictive and/or psychiatric disorders that may be present. We connect the dots and speak with other physicians, pharmacists, physical therapists, counselors, interventional anesthesiologists, acupuncturists, and concerned others to be sure we're all on the same page. The team at our clinic has witnessed the transformation of patients whose lives were severely impacted by chronic pain.

Pamela, a thirty-three-year-old woman with severe peripheral **neuropathy** and pain related to hepatitis C and AIDS, welcomed our approach, noting that she was relieved to learn we were not the kind of clinic that simply "threw pills" at her. She said that had never worked for her before.

A Day without Pain describes in detail many of the successful approaches that work in chronic pain treatment, placing a very strong emphasis not only on physical recovery and reduction of pain, but also on emotional, behavioral, and spiritual recovery. It is imperative to establish an environment where it is safe for patients to discuss their painful histories so that trust can be developed and grow.

Clinicians must work from a knowledgeable and compassionate mind-set and must be constantly vigilant about being empathetic, thus eliciting secondary gains from patients. Patients must be held strictly accountable to signed agreements. They have to learn about chronic pain syndrome and accept their roles in their recovery. They have to move their bodies from their poor conditioning to a state of much higher functioning.

In our clinic, we cheer patients on and continuously support and acknowledge small gains. We remind patients that it took a long time to get to their current place and that recovery is a process that takes time. We don't just look at pain relief. We view recovery in a much broader context. We scrutinize a patient's *functioning* with regard to life, mood, energy, spirituality, relationships, etc.

Our patients express gratitude that they are able to move from a "victim-stance," where they held onto their pain, to a position of taking back their lives.

Elizabeth is a forty-six-year-old woman who experienced early childhood abuse and came to us after suffering from migraine headaches and shoulder pain for twenty years. She had a history of chemical dependency and was already working a twelve-step recovery program. She said when she started treatment she had never heard the phrase "pain *management* program." She entered treatment with the notion that it was a "pain get rid of it" program. The turning point for Elizabeth was when she invited the pain in and faced it rather than running away from it. She was no longer a victim of chronic pain.

Finally, just as it's emphasized in *A Day without Pain*, we must encourage those who are struggling with chronic pain to never give up. We have seen so many lives change as a result of hard work. We believe in recovery and feel grateful to work with those suffering from chronic pain. For patients, we remain hopeful that functioning, mood, and pain can improve. There is help for professionals, families, and friends who are helplessly watching those in pain decline. We remain hopeful. We hope you will, too.

Barry M. Rosen, MD (1948–2009)
Andrea M. Wilcox, RN, MS, NP
San Mateo Medical Center Pain Clinic

PREFACE TO THE FIRST EDITION

"When it is dark enough, you can see the stars."

Ralph Waldo Emerson

This book is the culmination of several years working with people with chronic pain. In addition, it's the product of five years of my own journey with chronic pain. My bones have been creaky for a while, but one spring afternoon I simply bent forward and something "popped," and my life hasn't been the same since.

Many doctors and therapists have different theories as to what happened that day, but suffice it to say, I couldn't walk well or stand up straight, and my sleep was quite disturbed. I remained relatively functional, working, visiting with friends, traveling, and sleeping somewhat, but I never was pain-free. Usually the pain was just enough to aggravate, not incapacitate me. In my work lecturing is frequent, and by the forty-five-minute mark I would be in severe discomfort, which impeded my ability to concentrate.

Diagnostically, I went through the gamut; after all, I'm a doctor, for goodness' sake! I should know what's going on, and I have friends and colleagues who were all too eager to help.

My x-rays showed arthritis of the spine. Big deal. That's well expected in a fifty-something-year-old active man. I'd been in a few car accidents earlier in my life and had tweaked my back and neck, but never anything like this. An MRI showed a bulging disc on the left (the side of my discomfort at L 4-5 level) with no impingement of the nerve—a possible, but not likely, cause of my pain. The right side of the same disc showed a significant tear, but did not correlate with my symptoms. There also were ratty changes on the rest of my spine that would make a grown man weep and worry, which I did continuously and increasingly.

Therapeutically, I availed myself of a lot of different techniques that I read, heard, or knew about from my travels as a doctor. I consulted with chiropractors, acupuncturists, massage therapists, physical therapists, physicians, and finally a pain doctor who attempted a number of procedures including epidurals and facet joint injections with nerve **ablation**. I was twisted, poked with needles (large and small), odd substances were injected into my tissues, like steroids, phenol, and a variety of remedies from a doctor who did **prolotherapy**. My neck, hips, and sacroiliac joints were stretched and adjusted. My soft tissues were scraped with **Graston devices** and my sympathetic nervous system was down-regulated with **Primal Reflex Release Technique (PRRT)**. Some things helped for a short while, but frankly, the pain remained about the same. I got angrier, more frustrated, and a bit depressed.

Most of my frustration was that I couldn't exercise as I had previously. Walking was painful; hiking in the mountains was abandoned; swimming aggravated my shoulder (another story for another time); and standing became more troublesome. Running was totally out of the question. Yoga was doable, but my teacher, Veronica, needed to modify the class for me. I gained some weight and suffered with the inactivity.

Much as I hate to admit it, in some odd way, the pain I was experiencing and the consequences of having that pain served a function in my life. Actually, the pain had some surprising advantages for me. I didn't realize it at the time, but because of my pain I didn't have to exercise. I had a great excuse to sit around and watch TV, and, of course I had to eat while I was watching TV, which gave me an acceptable excuse for gaining weight. After all, I was in pain. In most of my conversations with friends and family, the opening line usually was "How's your back?" A well-timed groan or moan, more often than not, elicited the sought-after sympathetic "poor Melly . . ."

Now at the time, if you told me that any of this served me, I would have slugged you. After all, I was hurting, frustrated, furious, and miserable a good part of the time. I felt helpless, powerless, and hopeless. How could anyone suggest I was benefiting from my pain? Thankfully, not a soul *dared* to make such a suggestion. Without question this would have been a good reason to bite some heads off. I needed an excuse to yell and scream. As long as I stayed angry, my muscles stayed tight. The harder I tried to be powerful and overcome the pain, the more powerless and in pain I was. The more I resisted, the worse I hurt.

Today my pain is still there, but it is much less. What changed? My attitude. I experience my pain in an entirely different way. I got tired of the pain, of complaining, and of being miserable. I realized that my identity was my back pain, and I had become locked in the cycle of the futile search for the freedom from suffering. By my resisting, paradoxically, the hurt got worse. I learned to stop fighting and judging the pain. And, lo and behold, it disappeared—often for days at a time.

One of the insights I gained was that I was experiencing something known as secondary gain. In other words, I was gaining something (attention, sympathy, support, an excuse for my inactivity) from my negative or maladaptive behaviors. Furthermore, as I gave up my resistance, I found freedom.

I persisted with exercise and found a trainer who stretched me consistently. A consult with Sasha—a body worker, chiropractor, and spiritual healer—revealed many things, most importantly that I rotated my right foot outward when I walked or jogged, resulting in a pounding effect on my left side. He released (most painfully, I might add) some well-worn adhesions and knots in my back and shoulders while I shouted at the top of my lungs. I continued with yoga and added a daily walk with my dogs that reaped the benefits of my increased exercise tolerance. I also started to wear magnets in my shoes and on my back, which produced a sensation of heat and increased energy, as well as pain relief.

Just as important was my ongoing work at Las Vegas Recovery Center (LVRC) (see appendix) and writing this book. Clients at the center showed me their courage to persevere to an end that they couldn't imagine was real—true reduction in pain. I watched as they practiced the techniques described in this book including mindfulness, distraction, stretching, yoga, Pilates, Chi Kung, reiki, acupuncture, physical therapy, and attitude adjustment through group and individual therapy. As a part of the excellent team at LVRC, I was able to impart knowledge and experience, and by doing so learned some of my own lessons while I was teaching. I found the clients and their struggles helped me understand my own.

When I was busy and engaged, I had *no pain*. When my back started to throb, it was *always* because I was stressed or anxious about something. I sent positive energy into my pain rather than disdain and anger. I looked directly at the pain and it dissolved, as did the anger and fear. Because of my knowledge and personal recovery, I never took an opioid to relieve the pain. So, thankfully, I didn't need to contend with the negative effects opioids can cause. I developed a much more positive grip on my discomfort (it was down to a one or two on a ten-point scale for the most part by this time), and if it was there, I didn't fight against it, but simply saw that it was there and observed it with interest and curiosity. "Hmm, my pain has increased; I wonder what that's about?" I did this after months of practice, with increasingly positive effects. I did not suffer, and the pain was pretty much gone.

So as of today, I can say that I have a bit of pain, sometimes more than other times, but it's markedly reduced and very different than it used to be. Many times I find I have spent *A Day without Pain,* which is what I hope you will discover by reading this book.

ACKNOWLEDGMENTS

Thanks:

To the dedicated professionals at Las Vegas Recovery Center/Central Recovery Treatment: Stuart Smith, Brad Greenstein, Kristine and George Gatski, Debbie Champine, Joni Baumgart, Mary Jo Granieri, Matt Simo, Sandra Michael, Lynette Greenstein, Carline Allen, Teri Szabo, Sarah Day, Stephanie Laurent, Kim O'Donnell, Josh Koop, Jan Alberti, Larry Mendoza, Peter Perez, Pete Rappenecker, Bill Peiffer, Rich Bakir, DC, and all the managers, counselors, nurses, clinical associates, recovery technicians, and support staff.

Especially to John Lanzillotta, physician assistant extraordinaire, an excellent peer and colleague whether the topic is hypertension or mindfulness, diabetes or compassion. I couldn't do my work without him.

To my friend and colleague, Claudia Black, Ph.D., for the foreword to this second edition and for the endless hours of consulting, collaboration, and laughs.

To Amy Pitt, for her loving support and for reading the manuscript.

To Logan Smith, for preparation of the appendix.

To Eleanor and Phil Pohl and Denny Kay, who taught me about caring and compassion.

To my most supportive friends and family: Larry, Jackie, and Vida Pohl, Lisa and Oron Nadiv and Orion Hindawi, Kevin Kelly, Kekau Rosehill, Gary Schroeder, Greg Shay, Mikey Chambers, Jim Anderson, D Meyerson, Jerry Cade, Tilak Fernando, Kenny Butler, Gary Hamman, Paul Groce, Laura Fitzsimmons, John and Myk Lambrose, Kathy and Scott Dugan, Lynne and Rob Hunter, Irene Kay, Uncle Jack Pohl, Veronica Torres, Deanna and Dan Shiode, Sharon and Joe Cruse, Josephine and Jim Shakespeare, Mike Walas, Cindy West, Mark Lichtenstein, Nancy Sherman, Jay Beadle, Ginger Maiman, Lisa Jones, and Hugh Anderson.

To my professional colleagues and friends: the late Barry Rosen, MD, whom I miss very much, and Andrea Wilcox, RN, MS, NP, for writing the foreword to the first edition; Jodie Trafton, Ph.D.; Jim Tracy, DDS; Harry L. Haroutunian, MD; Herb Malinoff, MD; Howard Heit, MD; Cardwell C. Nuckols, MA, Ph.D.; John C. Friel, Ph.D.; and Ken Richardson, LISAC, CADC.

To Pema Chödrön, Thich Nhat Hanh, the Dalai Lama, and Jon Kabat-Zinn, whose lives and work I admire beyond words.

To all the folks at HCI.

To the therapists and doctors who stuck with me and saw me through my own personal journey toward a day without pain, especially Scott Pensivy; Will Allen; Mike McKenna, MD; Christian; Sasha; and Pierre.

To my editor, colleague, and friend, Nancy Schenck, a rigorous taskmaster who made the process a blast; and

To the CRP staff, especially Daniel Kaelin for editorial support and Patrick Hughes for marketing insights.

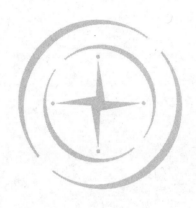

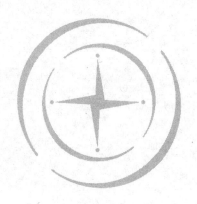

CHAPTER **1**

What Is Pain?

*"No kind of sensation is keener and
more active than that of pain,
its impressions are unmistakable."*

The Marquis de Sade

What is pain? What are the first words that come to mind when you think of pain? Is it sharp, aching, piercing, throbbing, relentless, stabbing, or is it aggravating, frightening, disabling, annoying, depressing? Each of us has a different and unique experience of pain—it is a combined experience that is both sensory and emotional. As with any experience, pain changes from moment to moment. Pain is the synthesis of myriad bits of information coming from within and without each of our bodies.

Pain is a necessary part of everyone's life. Why? Well, consider the following condition and the resulting consequences. Leprosy or Hansen's disease is a condition people develop that robs them of the ability to experience pain. Medical science has learned that the microorganism that causes leprosy infects the nervous system, resulting in the deterioration of the nerves with an ensuing inability to feel. The net result of such a condition is that because they can't feel anything, people with leprosy injure themselves without realizing it. Further injury thus results, and after a series of injuries over many years, these patients lose limbs and suffer irreparable harm, simply because they can't feel pain. This phenomenon is described eloquently in a book by Brand and Yancey called *Pain: The Gift Nobody Wants*.

So if pain is necessary, why do we become miserable when it doesn't resolve? There are two kinds of pain: acute and chronic. First, let's look at acute pain. Acute pain is a warning system; it tells us there is a problem somewhere. Then we do something about the problem, like withdraw from the flame, limp on a sore ankle, or remove the needle that's sticking in our finger. As with an alarm clock, we wake up and can turn off the buzzing. Similarly, with acute pain, as the body heals, the signal (pain, aching, throbbing, cramping) subsides and does not recur.

With chronic pain, the story is totally different.

Let's start with ten questions and answers about chronic pain.

Ten Questions About Pain

1 Why does pain exist? What function does it serve?
Pain exists to protect us from injury and, if we are injured, it protects us from further damage.

2 What is the difference between acute and chronic pain?
"The only thing acute and chronic pain have in common is the word 'pain.'" Acute pain ends when the body heals and the need for the pain is gone. Chronic pain never ends: The alarm clock goes off and continues to buzz—it annoys, detracts from life, irritates, frustrates, and *doesn't go away.*

3 What part of pain is associated with emotions? What percentage of chronic pain is emotional?
In my clinical practice, I have found that 80 percent or more of the experience of chronic pain is emotional.

4 Why won't the pain just go away?
The brain and the nervous system have changed, and they won't change back easily—not that they *can't* change back. A single-lane road becomes a four-lane highway, nerves are sensitized and their threshold for firing is lower, or they fire spontaneously and the nervous system's ability to down-regulate or turn off the pain signal is diminished.

5 What makes pain worse? Better?

Pain intensifiers include fear, anger, sadness, loneliness, and guilt. Distraction, movement, breathing, relaxing, and accepting make pain better.

6 Will I ever be free of pain?

Perhaps not free of pain, but certainly better able to have less pain at times and to accept pain when it occurs. You often don't notice the times when you get temporary relief from the pain if you are simply focused on how bad it is.

7 Why do I have to do things that hurt in order to get better?

The fear-avoidance cycle consists of not moving because it hurts. This results in being less able to move over time—movement causes more pain, and on and on. The solution is to move and stretch, despite the discomfort that eventually results in better mobility and improved self-efficacy. Stretching and increased movement correlate with lower pain levels.

8 How does chronic pain affect my family?

As it affects every aspect of your life, it affects every aspect of theirs: self-esteem and self-worth, satisfaction with life, emotions, sense of well-being. In other words, they feel your pain!

9 How can I get better from chronic pain?

The first step in getting better is to let go of the desire/need to be pain-free. Next, become willing to see that the emotional nature of your suffering is the way out for you. Work around the edges of the pain. Take responsibility for your actions with respect to functioning and medication use.

10 Why do I hold on to my pain?

You hold on to your pain for a variety of reasons. These relate to secondary gain, a typically unconscious driver of your discomfort—subtle benefits you achieve that drive you toward having more pain. These include not having to participate in activities, having an excuse to withdraw, allowing you to avoid emotions, and justification for taking medications.

Meet Paul

Paul was a vibrant, healthy, and athletic young man. He grew up in the Midwest playing a variety of sports and excelling at all of them. He was self-assured and charismatic. He graduated from college and then law school and was first in his class. He was well-liked and sought after for projects and parties. In every way, he was a golden boy. He dated many beautiful girls and then women and eventually entered a relationship with Lila, who had been a model in college and was working in a high-end fashion design office when they met. It was lust at first sight, and it eventually grew into a deep romance that led to marriage. They were a great-looking couple whom everyone wanted to be like and hang with.

After graduating from law school, Paul joined a high-powered corporate law firm and took to it immediately like a duck to water. Late hours of consuming work and client meetings with fine food and wine eventually led to tension at home. Lila was pregnant with their first child, and as her shape changed, so did her disposition. She felt violated and robbed of her looks, and was equally annoyed that her husband was never home. When he would finally arrive in their bed, he usually was exhausted and smelled of smoke and booze. This not only offended Lila, but made her feel nauseous. Feeling confused and sometimes hopeless, she would complain to her friends and family, "Where is the love we used to feel for each other?" More often than not, when she tried to talk with Paul, she had the distinct impression that he barely listened.

Eventually she broke down with Paul and told him how unhappy she was—always waiting for him to come home, frustrated that their relationship was suffering because of the demands of his job, and seriously concerned about his drinking. He dismissed her and her concerns with a round of "Come on, Lila, stop being such a prima donna. I have to be at these business functions. Besides, I work all day and I'm simply blowing off steam. This is what is expected of me." They grew apart and talked of separation, but the birth of their son silenced the discussion for a while. After the accident, everything changed.

Paul was driving home late at night after an eighteen-hour day and a dinner replete with wine and cigars. He would later learn that his blood alcohol level was 0.14, well over the legal limit of 0.08. He crashed into another car. In fact, he didn't even remember getting into his car. Paul's back and pelvis were fractured, and he learned that the driver of the other car was killed on impact.

When Paul regained consciousness, he was told the whole truth—he had killed a twenty-year-old woman. He was devastated by this news. In addition, he had totaled his car, crushed his pelvis and several discs in his back, and fractured his femur, and he was charged with DUI. His employer was holding his job, but his continued employment with the firm had become tenuous. While the firm valued his hard-driving nature, it had little stomach for scandal, and his prospects for returning to work were guarded at best. Lila was there at his bedside when he awoke in the most excruciating pain he had ever felt. He'd been sacked in football many times and broke a leg skiing years ago, but he had never experienced anything like this. "It feels like my leg is being dragged through my gut and taking my soul with it." He was a man of good conscience, and knowing his negligence was the cause of the accident overwhelmed him in a sea of unrelenting physical and emotional agony, relieved only by the increasing doses of morphine he was able to inject into himself via the pump attached to his arm.

He was charged with DUI, though not manslaughter. During the investigation into the accident, it was discovered that the accelerator had actually jammed that night due to a mechanical defect in the vehicle, resulting in his inability to stop the car. The contribution of his blood alcohol level was weighed, as was his physical condition and general state of disability. The fact that he was intoxicated worked against him and his defense. His former standing as a well-respected lawyer resulted, ultimately, in the other charges being dropped. But not for the girl's family, who held him accountable before God. Likewise, Paul held himself accountable and was consumed with remorse and shame.

Months passed. After six operations, Paul could finally walk with a limp, though he preferred to stay in bed. His firm finally fired him when they realized he wasn't coming back from the accident—physically or emotionally. Paul had changed after the crash that had taken another life, destroyed two families, and left him broken in body and in spirit. His pain was unrelenting, fueled by crushed nerve fibers, swollen joints, and guilt, as well as sorrow for everything he had lost. That made everything worse. Rather than physical therapy, he chose the mindlessness of TV talk shows. It hurt too much to move, so he didn't as he zoned out with a click of the remote control. He withdrew even more from Lila and took little joy in their son, William, as he grew through his milestones. Paul was filled with self-pity and oxycodone—an explosive combination.

What Paul had developed was the phenomenon known as chronic pain. What he would learn, and what I will discuss in this book, is that chronic pain is an experience that involves physical, emotional, mental, and spiritual components. At first, it signals that something is wrong and activates the body's "alert" system, telling you, "You'd better do something about the nail that is sticking in your finger. Take it out!"

For people in chronic pain, life can become an unpleasant grind, filled with negative messages from a nervous system gone haywire. Whether from cancer, from **fibromyalgia**, from back, leg, and hip problems, or from amputation, chemotherapy, diabetes, or hundreds of other causes, when we are in pain we can become consumed. Suddenly, we no longer merely live with pain; we become dominated by the sensations that depend in large measure on who is describing the feeling. These sensations bombard us, robbing us of comfort and well-being.

There are a number of scales by which to assess chronic pain. The simplest one is "On a scale of one to ten, rate your pain." Ten is the worst pain ever, and one is barely any pain. Obviously, this scale is quite subjective and gives only one number to use. The McGill Pain Questionnaire (see Table 1) offers a range of emotional and physical characteristics of pain, each of which you can rate as "none," "mild," "moderate," or "severe." I will also discuss the Pain Outcomes Profile (POP) in the Appendix.

Many Faces of Pain

Pain is universal. It has been experienced by every human who has ever walked the Earth. In the records of every civilization whose writings we can decipher, including those from thousands of years BC, there are descriptions of pain and how pain has been treated. For instance, to treat a painful back, the ancient Egyptians alternated the use of meat and honey, while the Greeks used traction and laying of the patient on a heated slab of marble. Early Greeks and Romans believed that the brain played a role

Table 1

SHORT-FORM McGILL PAIN QUESTIONNAIRE

RONALD MELZACK

PATIENT'S NAME _____ DATE _____

	NONE	MILD	MODERATE	SEVERE
THROBBING	0 _____	1 _____	2 _____	3 _____
SHOOTING	0 _____	1 _____	2 _____	3 _____
STABBING	0 _____	1 _____	2 _____	3 _____
SHARP	0 _____	1 _____	2 _____	3 _____
CRAMPING	0 _____	1 _____	2 _____	3 _____
GNAWING	0 _____	1 _____	2 _____	3 _____
HOT-BURNING	0 _____	1 _____	2 _____	3 _____
ACHING	0 _____	1 _____	2 _____	3 _____
HEAVY	0 _____	1 _____	2 _____	3 _____
TENDER	0 _____	1 _____	2 _____	3 _____
SPLITTING	0 _____	1 _____	2 _____	3 _____
TIRING-EXHAUSTING	0 _____	1 _____	2 _____	3 _____
SICKENING	0 _____	1 _____	2 _____	3 _____
FEARFUL	0 _____	1 _____	2 _____	3 _____
PUNISHING-CRUEL	0 _____	1 _____	2 _____	3 _____

NO PAIN |———————————————————| WORST POSSIBLE PAIN

PPI

0	NO PAIN	_____
1	MILD	_____
2	DISCOMFORTING	_____
3	DISTRESSING	_____
4	HORRIBLE	_____
5	EXCRUCIATING	_____

© R. MELZACK, 1984

in the perception of pain. A Babylonian day tablet, estimated to be over 4,000 years old, mentioned the use of henbane, a poisonous herb native to Europe and Asia, to treat pain. Acupuncture and Ayurveda are two of the earliest medical practices, and they come from China and India, respectively. The first record of acupuncture is found in the 4,700-year-old *Huang Di Neijing* (*Yellow Emperor's Classic of Internal Medicine*). This is said to be the oldest medical textbook in the world. Ayurveda literally means "the science of life" and focuses on the integration and balance of the body, mind, and spirit. As early as the nineteenth century, **opioids** such as morphine were used to reduce pain. Many of these techniques and interventions are in use today to treat pain.

> *While pain is universal, the experience of pain is quite subjective, since what every individual feels when in pain is unique to that individual.*

While pain is universal, the experience of pain is quite subjective, since what every individual feels when in pain is unique to that individual. As Brand and Yancey state in *Pain: The Gift Nobody Wants*, "Few experiences in life are more universal than pain, which flows like lava beneath the crust of daily life." How each of us interprets and reacts to a painful stimulus is incredibly complex and involves many factors, including age, gender, ethnicity, culture, religion, environment, attitudes, stereotypes, and social influences. For example, as is typical in many a Jewish household, complaining was part and parcel of everyday life for me and my family. "Kvetching" was a common way to express suffering in my house. In Asian and certain African cultures, on the other hand, it is common to take a stoic attitude (or maintain a stiff upper lip) with barely a whimper for a woman giving birth or when someone is injured. Being "tough" is regarded as an asset in the military and in various households steeped in the tradition of "manning up."

As we mature, we learn what pain means to us through our personal experiences. The pain experience is so varied that it's possible to get many different descriptions of pain from people exposed to identical pain-inducing stimuli. Furthermore, you may have different perceptions of identical stimuli depending on the time of day, temperature, circumstances (where you are and what you are doing), how much sleep you got last night, weather conditions, and so forth. For Paul, his pain was much worse on the weekends, when Lila was around and the baby was crying or making noise so that he couldn't sleep. On cold, rainy days, his leg ached much worse than on warm, sunny days. And on the day his parents visited, his level of pain shot through the roof. Conversely, if he was able to get out to an engaging movie or if Lila surprised him with pizza from his favorite restaurant, his pain level subsided temporarily.

Pain is that feeling or group of feelings you experience when you smash your thumb, have a heart attack, get a splinter, bump your head, get run over by a car, touch a hot stove, cut off a finger, knock out a tooth, get shot, stub a toe, pick up something too heavy, get poked in the eye with a stick, experience childbirth, or wake up after surgery. And each of these types of pain will feel quite different to each of you. Pain is a perception rather than just a sensation. If this is true, let's look at where we experience perception. It is in our brain—more specifically, our mind. The emotional effect on our perceptions occurs in the **limbic system** (described in Chapter Three). Emotions play a large role in our experience of pain and suffering. For example, pain is worse when we are depressed. This is because a depressed brain actually *feels* more pain.

You probably could fill in many more examples. In fact, take a few minutes to jot down some of the pain experiences you've had.

Acute and Chronic Pain

As I've already discussed, there are two types of pain, acute and chronic. Acute pain is the feeling you get when you damage your body—burn a finger, break an arm, stub a toe, twist an ankle, or bump your head. It's a signal that something is wrong and needs attention. It is time-limited and responds to medication or other therapies, and eventually just subsides over time as the body heals. A headache or stomachache or broken bone or sprained ankle are examples of acute pain. Acute pain is generally relieved once the cause has been addressed and the process has resolved, even though it may take weeks or even months for the pain to finally end.

Acute pain does not last longer than six months. It ends when the body no longer "needs" it. For Paul, the leg he broke while skiing healed and the pain in that limb resolved for good. Acute pain is part of the body's defense system, which, when triggered, brings about physical and mental behaviors to try to end the pain-causing experience and to protect the body, giving it a chance to heal. Acute pain is based in an extremely effective educational system. Once you experience pain in a given situation, it is unlikely that you will actively seek to repeat the painful situation. For example, you need only burn your hand once on a hot stove to learn not to touch a hot stove.

How We Feel Pain

At its most basic level, pain is a word that describes discomfort. That discomfort generally is the result of some action or event that has occurred in your world, which you notice when nerve cells or **neurons** in your body carry their message to your brain via the spinal cord. In short, if you get stuck with a nail in your finger, the neurons of the finger start to fire and transmit a signal up the spinal column to the brain. The spinal column is a relay station.

Pain is an adaptive, useful response, telling you to guard sore or damaged tissue and give it time to heal. It's a component of your alert or early-warning system. Special nerve cells called **nociceptors** are the neurons that sense pain in animals—including humans. The primary home for neurons is the spinal cord, and from there they connect to every part and organ of the human body. When these nerve fibers are excited by a painful stimulus message, they transmit the message to the brain, which releases a flood of chemicals called **neurotransmitters**. In Paul's case, much of the pain he first experienced when he broke his leg was the result of the stimulation of nociceptors, the specialized nerves that react to disruption of the bone and soft tissues related to the injury. The body has a graded response to the damage—that is, the more severe the problem, the more intense the acute pain.

Nociceptors react to temperatures (hot or cold), pressure, and a variety of chemicals released by cells close to the source of pain. Nociceptors are able to send information to the brain that pinpoints the location, the nature, and the intensity of the pain. In general, if the pain is severe (the tissue damage substantial), the body transmits the feeling rapidly to the brain. Less severe pain (generally indicating less tissue damage) is processed or transmitted less rapidly over a different set of nerve fibers. The initial response of the pain system results in a feeling or perception in the damaged tissue that might evoke an "ouch" and the desire to escape the cause of the discomfort. The intensity of the pain perception also corresponds to the magnitude of the tissue damage or seriousness of the pain. For example, being crushed under a fifty-pound weight hurts more than being stung by a bee.

Chronic Pain

Chronic pain is entirely different from acute pain. The late Dr. Barry Rosen, an addiction specialist and former medical director of the San Mateo Medical Center Pain Clinic in California, used to say, "The only thing acute pain and chronic pain have in common is the word 'pain.'" Chronic pain refers to pain that continues after an acute injury heals or after the passing of a period of time that should allow for healing. In the case of chronic pain, the discomfort persists for six months or longer. Examples are cancer pain, pain related to a persistent or degenerative disease, and long-term pain from unidentifiable causes. Unrelieved pain eventually becomes chronic. Chronic pain is a complex disorder that lasts for more than six months, has outlived its usefulness, and is much more complicated than acute pain. It is a disease process with biological, mental, emotional, and spiritual components. In many cases, the cause(s) of chronic pain cannot be determined, and the pain is resistant to medical treatment. Chronic pain from causes other than cancer is referred to as chronic nonmalignant pain or chronic noncancer pain (CNCP). Most often, this involves damage to the central and peripheral nervous systems.

Neuropathic pain refers to damage or injury to the nerve fibers themselves that results in misfiring of the nerves. Some common causes of neuropathic pain are nerve damage from alcohol toxicity, vitamin deficiencies, amputation (phantom limb syndrome), chemotherapy, diabetes, infections, HIV or AIDS, multiple sclerosis, sciatica, and herpes zoster (shingles), to name just a few. Often there is no obvious cause for neuropathic pain, as is also the case with **trigeminal neuralgia**.

Neuropathic pain has what are called "positive symptoms," referring to the presence of abnormal sensations such as heat, electric shock, shooting, stabbing, crawling, itching, or burning. Neuropathic pain may also include negative symptoms or the absence of feeling, specifically numbness, which can be very disconcerting.

Central pain is a condition where the brain and nervous system are altered, resulting in *feeling* more pain. Central pain includes **allodynia**, which is pain from a stimulus that does not ordinarily cause pain, and **hyperalgesia**, which is pain that is much more intense than it should be—an exaggeration or distortion of the pain than would normally be expected. An example of allodynia is the excruciating pain caused by the light touch of clothing to the skin after severe sunburn. Hyperalgesia can result from a simple pinprick to the finger, causing sharp, stabbing pain that feels out of proportion to the pinprick. Hyperalgesia also can be felt all over the body and may be caused by opioid painkillers (see page 55).

Central pain occurs due to **sensitization** of the brain and nervous system. This happens when your nervous system magnifies and warps the feeling of pain, turning an already painful condition into something much worse. Sensitization may affect all of your pain-processing areas, including the nociceptors, spinal column, and thought-processing centers. Central pain is often misunderstood—thought to be less "real"—since when this occurs chronic pain becomes associated with emotional and psychological suffering, including a host of emotions such as depression, anger, stress, fear, frustration, hopelessness, and rage. Though it seems to be made up or imagined, it is not—it's as real as any other kind of chronic pain. The problem with central pain is that the intensity of the pain signal in the brain is turned up on high.

Stephen Colameco, MD, M.Ed., assistant clinical professor in the Department of Family Medicine, University of Medicine and Dentistry of New Jersey–School of Osteopathic Medicine, explains in *12 Steps for Those Afflicted with Chronic Pain:* "Chronic pain seems purposeless. Chronic pain is disabling because it takes away the ability to perform activities that others consider routine. Those with chronic pain are often irritable and depressed or overly dependent on others. They are left wondering why they are in pain when others are not, what they might have done to deserve this fate."

What's Next?

Chronic pain is complex, with many different layers that affect your thoughts, emotions, body, and spirit. It can be relentless, and poses a very real threat to living a full and vigorous life. In this book I will discuss many aspects of pain, including the many characteristics of chronic pain. You will discover information about the brain, medications used to treat pain, addiction, feelings/emotions, effects of chronic pain on families, various methods of treatment, and spirituality. The following chapters will also explore and explain the complicated nature of chronic pain. I will offer comprehensive solutions so that you can replace a self-image of disability and pain with one of wellness, balance, and restored function. This book is meant to be informative, as well as a resource with avenues to provide a perspective about chronic pain for your family and for you. In my work with those with chronic pain, I am always amazed at the resilience and strength of their ability, over time and with proper treatment, to improve and shine through their pain experience. *A Day without Pain* is here to help you live with the daunting problem and amazing opportunity called pain.

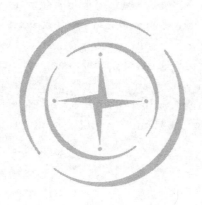

CHAPTER 2

Chronic Pain Never Goes Away

"Under such torments, the temper changes,
the most amiable grow irritable,
the bravest soldier becomes a coward..."

Dr. S. Weir Mitchell

There is no one representative face of pain. It is the scraped knee of a young child or the tumor pressing on the spine of her grandfather; it is her mother in labor, shouting for relief, anticipating the arrival of a new life; and it is the countless variations of human conditions we may experience throughout life. Chronic pain is persistent back pain after an injury, cancer, persistent headaches, heart problems, shortness of breath, scar tissue from surgery, fibromyalgia, irritable bowel syndrome, carpal tunnel syndrome, or **complex regional pain syndrome** (formerly called **reflex sympathetic dystrophy/causalgia**). It is impossible to put "a face" on chronic pain because it is millions of faces, all different, all distinctive. Nevertheless, while chronic pain is experienced differently by every individual, it is important to understand that those in chronic pain are tied together with certain commonalities.

Chronic pain affects so many of us that we would need a long list of the types of people who are affected to adequately describe all the variations. And just as the face of chronic pain is everyone yet no single one, so, too, are their paths unique in leading to the consequences of chronic pain for every individual.

Chronic pain is hundreds of different conditions. An exhaustive list would take up the rest of this book, but here are several examples of chronic pain:

- Back, neck, and joint pain, which can result from tension, muscle injury, nerve damage, disc disease, or arthritis.

- Burn pain, which continues after a burn wound has healed.

- Chronic pelvic pain, which refers to any pain in your pelvic region, including from tumors, infections, or scar tissue.

- Cancer pain, which can result from the growth of a tumor with pressure on nerves, treatment of the disease (chemotherapy or radiation treatments), or other effects of cancer on the body (blockage, organ damage, and so on).

- Infections that don't respond to treatment, and that can occur anywhere in the body.

- Chronic abdominal pain for which there may be no physical explanation or findings.

- Inflammatory bowel disease, ulcers, irritable bowel syndrome, colitis, Crohn's disease, or other intestinal problems.

- Bursitis, which can affect any joint, usually knees, shoulders, hips, elbows, or wrists.

- Head and facial pain, which can be caused by dental problems, temporomandibular joint (TMJ) disorder, trigeminal neuralgia, Ramsey Hunt syndrome (a painful rash around the ear that occurs when the varicella zoster (chicken pox) virus infects a nerve in the head) or other disorders affecting the nerves in the face, or chronic headaches, including migraines, cluster headaches, and tension headaches.

- Multiple sclerosis, which can cause numbness, aching, or pain.

- Angina or chest pain from heart disease.

- Uterine fibroid tumors, growths in the womb that can be associated with bleeding.

- Chronic obstructive pulmonary disease (COPD) or emphysema.

- Peripheral vascular disease (inadequate blood circulation to arms and legs).

- Ankylosing spondylitis, or severe arthritis with restriction of spinal movement.

- Pancreatitis, which is the inflammation of one of the most important digestive organs in the body.

- Myofascial pain syndromes, which result in painful trigger points in a person's muscles; fibromyalgia is characterized by tenderness in multiple areas of the body, widespread muscle pain, fatigue, and stiffness.

- Whiplash after an accident.

- Broken bones that have healed incompletely or in the wrong position.

This list is not complete, of course, but underscores the many diverse types of chronic pain.

Scope of the Problem

Chronic pain is one of the most significant, costly, and problematic issues facing America today. Tens of millions are afflicted; pain is the most frequent reason Americans seek medical attention. Approximately 24 percent of men and 27 percent of women in the United States—more than 76 million people—experience long-lasting, chronic pain that persists for months, years, decades, or a lifetime. Government agencies report that 22 percent of patients coming to a primary physician report being in pain; 83 million adults report that pain affects their participation in an activity; 6 million patients die in pain from cancer each year; and 25 percent of nursing home residents experience daily pain. Nearly 50 million are partially or completely disabled. Chronic pain causes more disability in the United States than cancer and heart disease combined.

More than $100 billion per year is spent on pain, and chronic pain costs the nation an additional $60 billion in lost productivity annually. That means the direct cost of chronic pain in the United States can be conservatively estimated to be more than $160 billion per year. These costs do not include the suffering experienced by those in pain and their families. It is believed that chronic pain is one of the most common causes of suicide. Despite all these staggering statistics, there still seems to be no ultimate solution to end chronic pain.

All pain is real

All pain is real, just as Paul's pain was real, despite there no longer being an obvious acute physical reason for its presence. His bones had healed, his back was fused, and his nerves conducted normally, according to **electromyography (EMG)** tests. But he still hurt—all day, every day. This is common for many who have chronic pain. There is not always a concrete and obvious reason for the pain, but it continues to disturb their well-being. For Paul, the pain signals in his now-healed pelvis and leg just kept firing, mistakenly signaling that something was still wrong, something still needed attention, despite the measures already taken to correct his problem. Unfortunately, Paul was in the same boat with many of you who have chronic pain.

Chronic Pain Syndrome

The sad truth about chronic pain is that it may eventually take over a person's life, as it did Paul's. It is a major challenge to health care providers because of its natural history, poor response to therapy, and often unclear causes. Paul faced this very dilemma. He suffered with chronic pain, abused prescription opioids, and felt unending remorse, sorrow, and overwhelming loneliness. He lost his job, his self-esteem, and whatever was meaningful in his life. Paul felt alone in the world and wanted to be left alone, all at the same time. Not only was he unable to do the things he once believed normal; his inability to "make people understand" about his pain isolated him even further. The extreme isolation Paul experienced is common for those in chronic pain.

Preoccupation with pain can lead to a vicious cycle in which the person enters a state of profound suffering. Paul could not sleep, and the next day's weariness led to irritability, despair, and more pain, which compounded the sleep problem, which led to more irritability, frustration, and anger. This situation was invariably made worse by his taking medications regularly and experiencing their inescapable side effects.

In way too many cases, chronic pain evolves into chronic pain syndrome (CPS), a constellation of several detectable symptoms and characteristics that occur together. The features include, but are not limited to:

- Pain that has lasted for more than six months.

- Feelings of depression, anger, worry, discouragement, irritability, and fear.

- Sleep difficulties.

- Monetary problems.

- Problems relating to others, causing significant disturbance in relationships.

- An inability to tolerate activities.

- Withdrawal from social activities.

- Inability to concentrate.

- Poor memory.

- A decrease in sexual activity or performance.

- A decrease in self-esteem.

- Secondary physical problems.

- Misuse of pain medications and/or alcohol.

- Avoiding work and leisure activities.

- Negative attitudes concerning everyday life.

This array of symptoms demonstrates well the emotional complexities that are an integral part of the experience of this type of pain. For Paul, and for millions more, chronic neuropathic and central pain resulted from damage to the nervous system. Neuropathic and central pain can be mild or can be so severe that it impacts every facet of life: sleep, work, mobility, relationships, enjoyment, and overall function.

It is probable that Paul's pain resulted from damage to the nerves in his spine that he suffered in the car accident prior to his first surgery. Paul's pain was also the result of a change in his brain, which began with his first injury but progressed well beyond that condition. Most people experiencing neuropathy complain of numbness, burning, tingling, muscle weakness, a "pins-and-needles" feeling, or, as with Paul, a combination of all of these. Paul's pain also involved his emotional responses to the pain, which magnified his suffering. Paul had central pain that caused him to really be in more pain than seemed "appropriate" to his surgeon and his pain doctor. "He should be better now. I've done everything I can for him," said the surgeon, in essence implying there was something else wrong with Paul. Lila couldn't help but think Paul exaggerated the amount of pain he was in to justify his taking of drugs.

There is no accurate and foolproof way to measure the intensity of a person's pain. There is no x-ray, magnetic resonance imaging (MRI), or other scan or test that will reliably reveal the amount of pain a person has. There is no scientific instrument that will precisely and reliably identify the type, duration, or exact origin of the pain; however, cutting-edge research is bringing us closer all the time. Doctors are even less able to comprehend and understand your suffering. Currently, physicians must rely on your description of what you are experiencing. So when Paul complained that his pain was an eight or nine on a ten-point scale, no one could refute his experience, and the medication dosages escalated accordingly.

How Acute Pain Becomes Chronic Pain

Like acute pain, chronic pain often begins with an injury. For unknown reasons, the injury or tissue damage doesn't heal as expected. Because of this, the nociceptors continue to fire as if there is damage that needs attention. With this unrelenting signal traveling up the spinal column to the brain, eventually the transmission circuits become more efficient at transmitting these signals—like a one-lane road becoming a four-lane highway. In other words, the bombarding of the circuits causes more transmission, with the net result being more pain. Furthermore, the number of neurotransmitters in the nervous system that cause pain (like **substance P, enkephalins,** and others) increases. Over time, the threshold for the nociceptors to fire is lowered. A less intense stimulus is needed to cause the nerve to discharge and send its signal.

We are left with a system that has changed to produce more pain than is necessary for protection. The pain signal just keeps firing, becoming an annoyance, an irritation, and ultimately, a source of misery.

Furthermore, there is a normal part of the nervous system that sends inhibitory signals down the spinal column, normally quelling pain that is unnecessary or bothersome. This is useful if you have pain that can't be dealt with. For example, if you sprain your ankle while running for a touchdown, your body is able to turn off the pain so you can complete the task. This type of signal is decreased as well, so with chronic pain, you are left with even more pain.

Understanding Chronic Pain

In order to more fully understand the complex nature of chronic pain, let's look at a model created by professionals to help explain the phenomenon. Historically, practitioners generally defined pain in biomedical terms. That is, chronic pain was believed to be dual in nature—of the mind and body. Traditionally, for those specialists it was explainable solely in biological or medical terms. The biomedical model of pain accepts that emotional and mental problems may result from chronic pain, but that the pain itself is entirely biological in origin and the most effective treatment for it is medical in nature. Real pain was "physical" and emotions were discounted, with patients labeled hypochondriacs or malingerers. This leaves millions out of luck, because let's face it, traditional medicine has failed more than helped when it comes to chronic pain.

Professionals used to think the emotional manifestations of pain were in some way less "real" than physical pain. People's emotional pain was called psychosomatic or, worse, they were labeled hypochondriacs. But where do emotions come from? They come from a complex interaction in the brain of electrical and chemical impulses, resulting in a cascade of nerves firing and chemicals being secreted—emotions are creations of the physical brain, just like pain.

> ### *Emotions are creations of*
> ### *the physical brain, just like pain.*

As my understanding of pain has grown, it has become clearer to me and others treating chronic pain, as well as to researchers, that pain is multidimensional. It involves our bodies, thoughts, emotions, and spirits. In *Pain Recovery: How to Find Balance and Reduce Suffering from Chronic Pain*, we write about attaining a healthy lifestyle by achieving balance in the whole person. This requires working with the physical (sensory) pain as well as your emotional responses and thoughts about the pain. People with chronic pain often become spiritually disconnected and will benefit from finding spiritual balance, regardless of their religious beliefs. As balance is achieved, you will be able to develop healthy relationships and take positive actions.

Cultural and Gender Influences on Chronic Pain

Cultural differences have an impact on the intensity of the pain you feel, how you describe the pain, your tolerance for pain, and how you cope with pain. Learning about pain takes place within a definite social context, which means the way you behave when you are in pain is a reflection of the culture in which you were raised. It has been shown that those from some cultures believe complaining is a sign of weakness, so they don't complain. Conversely, in other cultures (like mine—have I told you about my back pain?) complaining about pain is considered beneficial to the sufferer.

There are cultures that practice rituals in which incredibly painful activities are a part of daily life. For example, some African tribes initiate young males into adulthood by slicing their bodies literally thousands of times. The young men must endure the procedure silently, with virtually no reaction. Their feelings of pain and their reaction to it are heavily influenced by the culture in which it is being felt.

One Native American tribal culture once used a "sun dance" to initiate young males into adulthood. The tribal shaman would cut slits in the chests of initiates and then insert bone hooks into the slits. The young males were expected to hang by the hooks while looking at the sun until their flesh tore and they were free. This entire painful experience was to be endured in silence.

Some cultures encourage women to make noise during labor while others expect silence, a sort of "grin and bear it" attitude. Different societies have different expectations regarding labor pain. American women, for example, when compared with women from Holland, expect labor to be more painful and also anticipate receiving more pain medication. Some women in Asia deliver their children under acupuncture anesthesia. In addition, there are differences in the cultural expression of pain, such as wailing or crying.

Families play a very significant role in the development of the pain experience. Parents become role models as to how pain should be expressed and handled. Researchers have found that children from homes where a parent has chronic pain have significantly higher rates of pain problems. Families become a sounding board for pain perceptions. In some, such mechanisms can lead to behaviors that may have negative effects on the pain sufferers' lives. For example, some families stress the excessive use of bed rest to relieve pain, or the use of medications to "take away the pain" is encouraged. Pain is looked at as an unnecessary evil that should be banished at all costs. In many cases, both of these behaviors can actually lead to increased degrees of pain and disability later in life.

Gender is another important factor in how we feel pain. Men and women respond to pain differently, and in fact, they are affected differently by pain. The sex hormones estrogen and testosterone definitely play a role in this distinction, but psychology and culture account for some of the differences. Of the millions who live with chronic pain in the United States, women report experiencing pain more often and with greater intensity than men. On the other hand, researchers have found women are less likely to let pain control their lives. They are quicker to seek help for their pain, and they also are quicker to recover from pain. Studies have documented that the natural painkilling system in men and women is different. Additionally, gender can influence how one talks about and copes with pain.

Stereotypical roles of each gender in society help to influence their reactions to pain. For example, in most American cultures men are more apt to be discouraged from expressing their pain, and women encouraged to express theirs. There is a strong correlation of pain levels in twins with menstrual pain and with migraine, which points to a genetic component of pain.

In one animal study, it was found that morphine works differently in males and in females. Additionally, women may be more affected by a painful stimulus because women are more sensitive to threats. This probably relates to a maternal need to be alert to danger and protect their offspring. Women are far more likely to be in touch with their physical experiences, and they experience more anxiety and depression than men, both of which are linked to a higher level of pain or more intense pain.

Pain Teaches Us

A significant feature of chronic pain is emotional pain felt in the body. At its most basic level, you generally experience acute emotional pain for the same reasons you experience acute physical pain. Like feeling the burn from touching a hot stove tells you to stop touching it, emotional pain occurs so you will stop doing something, learn, and grow.

People feel emotional pain in reaction to traumatic events or situations, such as a car accident, divorce, death or loss of a loved one, emotional/physical/sexual abuse, or the onset of chronic physical pain. Research shows that the actual event is not the cause of emotional pain, but rather the way the person experiences and reacts to the event. This typically results in a pattern of recurrent responses; for example, fear, anxiety, and anger may be expressed as a headache.

In no way am I suggesting that the pain and suffering are not real. For example, as the doctors focused on Paul's back instead of addressing his grief, guilt, and anger, they ended up missing potential opportunities of successfully treating his chronic pain. This way of looking at pain will have important implications when I discuss treatment in Chapters Eight and Ten.

Meet Phyllis

Phyllis grew up in the Northeast in a nonreligious Christian family. Her mom was bedridden for weeks at a time with headaches and arthritis, and when she had her "monthly," she'd be out of commission for at least a week. As a youngster—well before puberty—Phyllis learned to prepare food for her father and younger brother. She was in charge and accepted the responsibility without question.

By the time Phyllis was twelve years old, her mom was in bed more than being up and around. Phyllis was the "woman of the house," and she took pride in this. It was a natural transition to the expanded role her father chose for her when he started creeping into her room late at night, fondling her and warning her to be quiet. "Don't disturb your poor sick mother," he would whisper. So she submitted to his increasingly aggressive sexual advances.

Early in her young life, Phyllis developed a painful, sick feeling in her gut—and in her soul. It was entangled with her shame about so many things. She felt responsible to care for her parents, and little by little she began to disappear into her pain. By the age of fifteen, Phyllis had begun to experience soreness in her joints and muscles, much like her mother and aunt. They had both been diagnosed with fibromyalgia, and Phyllis became convinced she had the same syndrome. Like them, she began taking a variety of substances, including Tylenol, aspirin, and Motrin. Eventually, she started "borrowing" her mother's prescription painkillers.

Phyllis used these medications to numb the gnawing emotional pain she felt every moment she was alive. She also felt furious and powerless toward her abusive father, while at the same time she was consumed with guilt over what she was sure would send her straight to hell. As with many abused children, Phyllis felt she had done something wrong and deserved punishment. In addition to her emotional pain, she found it was becoming harder and harder to ignore the aching in her shoulders, wrists, hips, and back.

She left the house for good at the age of sixteen. Her mother had been hospitalized for months and eventually died from ovarian cancer. Phyllis had no reason to stay. In fact, she needed to escape the now-nightly drunken advances from her father. She simply refused to put up with it another minute. She had met an older boy who introduced her to heroin and methamphetamine, and in no time she was hooked. She took off with him and hit the streets of Chicago in short order.

Mood Affects Pain

Mood is inextricably linked to the experience of pain. Depression is one of the most common components of CPS. Chronic pain and depression are irrevocably linked. CPS causes depression; depression increases pain. More than 30 percent of those with chronic pain also have clinical depression. At least 75 percent of those with depression also have pain. It has been proven that if you experience depression connected with CPS, you will experience more physical impairment because of the pain. And the more pain a person feels, the more likely it is that that person will have associated problems such as anxiety, sleeplessness, sadness, anger, and stress.

Standard symptoms of major depression include a persistently sad or "empty" mood; feelings of pessimism, hopelessness, helplessness, and worthlessness; fatigue or loss of interest in ordinary activities, including sex; sleep and eating disturbances; irritability, anger, increased crying, anxiety, and panic; difficulty concentrating, remembering, or making decisions; and thoughts of suicide and making suicide plans or attempts. Substance abuse is often associated with depression and certainly worsens the perception of pain.

Paul and Phyllis, like too many others, believed their feelings of hopelessness and helplessness were an inextricable part of their lot in life, a punishment for what they had done. Paul was constantly at odds with everyone and everything. He would become enraged with little provocation. Life was a continuous struggle—he just wanted to be left alone. There was no more joy, no more fun. There was only pain and suffering. If he took enough medications to block out reality, he was left in a virtual stupor until they wore off. Phyllis was a lost soul, functioning only in the world she created of drugs and sex.

As your physical pain symptoms increase, the amount and severity of psychological pain inevitably increase as well. Accepting that you are depressed in addition to being in pain, and treating your depression as well as your pain, can help reduce both. Trauma also predisposes a person to developing central pain. Phyllis had suffered sexual trauma since she was a little girl and was essentially set up for the misery of fibromyalgia, a form of central pain, and the drug addiction that followed. Her drug use fueled her depression and made the pain worse. The effects of Paul's accident had an impact on him both physically and emotionally. The traumas that Phyllis and Paul suffered caused the volume knob in their brains' pain centers to be turned way up.

That depression and pain are closely linked can be seen in the circuitry of the nervous system. In pain, communication between the body and brain goes both ways. Researchers have discovered that the areas of the brain that handle pain use some of the same neurotransmitters involved in mood, including serotonin, dopamine, and norepinephrine. Researchers are looking to the brain to unlock and understand depression. As we will see in the next chapter, exciting research on the brain has provided us with and expanded our understanding of chronic pain.

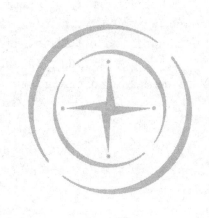

CHAPTER 3

No Brain, No Pain

*"If the brain were so simple we could understand it,
we would be so simple we couldn't."*

Dr. Lyall Watson*

In this chapter I will attempt to simplify the most complex organ in the body. There are more cells in the nervous system than there are stars in the universe, and each nerve cell has thousands of contacts with other neurons, totaling trillions of such connections.

First, I'll explain some of the different sections of the brain. Then I will describe some of the parts of the brain involved in feeling pain and how something painful gets from the site of origin of the pain to the inside of your head. Then I'll explain how scientists, using chemicals and scientific instruments, can actually see areas of the brain that are affected by pain. When you do something that hurts, the areas of the brain where you feel pain (the **thalamus**) "light up." Scientists have learned that emotions have an effect on pain because experiencing these emotions or feelings causes activation of the pain centers of the brain.

I'll then show you how changing the brain is not always something that merely happens to you, but also is something you can *cause* to happen. For example, some people prone to depression actually have changed their own brain's chemistry so they're not as likely to get depressed. Regular meditators have been shown to cause nerve cells to "sprout" in anticipation of forming new connections with other nerve cells. Studying and learning also result in the brain changing.

*Used with permission of Dr. Lyall Watson.

Finally, I'll tie it all together and discuss how the discovery of **plasticity** of the brain, or the brain's ability to change, has sparked a promise of exciting applications and treatments—the possibility that schizophrenics can improve their symptoms, that someone with Alzheimer's disease can slow or even stop the progression of the disease, and that those who have chronic pain can decrease their own level of pain and change some of the problems associated with it.

The brain is the most intricate and complex part of human anatomy. It regulates your heartbeat, breathing, blood pressure, and temperature. It allows you to sleep, dream, love, hate, fear, and laugh. It controls your sight, smell, taste, touch, and hearing. It allows you to walk, sit, stand, jump, crouch, stand on tiptoes, talk, and perform countless other activities. It is in your brain that you develop your personality and your mind. The brain weighs only three pounds, and it is the essence of your humanity.

And, most importantly for this discussion, the brain is the architect, mediator, and regulator of pain.

For much of history, scientists have been in the dark about the brain. In the last twenty years, however, improvements in neurological and behavioral science, better research techniques, and vastly superior medical and scientific machinery have finally allowed scientists and researchers to begin to understand the brain—to see and figure out how it functions.

Brain Basics 101

Scientists have learned much about the brain from people who have suffered strokes or other losses of function. They can correlate areas of the brain with functional losses and determine what those brain sections do. The brain can be divided into three parts, the **forebrain**, the **midbrain**, and the **hindbrain**. All three parts work together, but each has its own individual properties, according to the National Institute of Neurological Disorders and Stroke (NINDS), which conducts and supports scientific studies on the brain in the United States and around the world.

The hindbrain controls the body's vital involuntary functions, and includes the upper part of the spinal cord, the brain stem, and the **cerebellum**. The cerebellum regulates involuntary activities such as breathing, heartbeat, temperature control, and fluid balance. It also coordinates movement and is involved in learned activities such as when you hit a baseball or play a musical instrument. Just above the hindbrain is the midbrain, which controls some reflex actions, eye movements, other voluntary movements, and the vast array of emotions you feel. The midbrain also is charged with keeping the individual and species alive through various activities. The forebrain is the largest and most highly developed part of the brain; it consists of the **cerebrum,** or the **frontal lobes,** and the structures beneath.

Coating the surface of the cerebrum and the frontal lobes is a thin layer of tissue called the **cerebral** or **frontal cortex** (*cortex* means "bark" in Latin). Most of the information processing in the brain takes place in the cerebral cortex. When scientists and researchers talk about gray matter in the brain, they are talking about this thin layer. The cortex, NINDS explains, is gray because nerves in this area lack the insulation (**myelin**) that makes most other parts of the brain appear to be white.

Deep inside the brain are structures that act as gatekeepers between the spinal cord and the frontal lobes. These structures allow you to initiate movements without thinking; they determine your emotional state, and they modify your perceptions and responses depending on that state. It is this area of the brain that tells you to move your hand away from a hot stove when you've been burned. You do so without a thought or even a conscious awareness.

When the brain is in good physical shape it functions instantaneously, without you even thinking about it. But when problems occur, the results can be a slowing or breakdown of functions. Many severe illnesses may result. Some of the major disorders that happen when there is a brain problem include:

- Inherited diseases, e.g., Huntington's disease and muscular dystrophy.

- Developmental disorders, e.g., cerebral palsy.

- Degenerative diseases of adults, e.g., Parkinson's disease and Alzheimer's disease.

- Cerebrovascular diseases, e.g., strokes and aneurysms.

- Infectious diseases, e.g., AIDS and toxoplasmosis.

- Brain tumors and other malignancies.

- Trauma, e.g., spinal cord and head injuries.

Biology of Pain

Scientists have long understood that the feeling of pain is located in the brain; hence, "no brain, no pain." To understand the biology of pain, let's look at what happens when you get a nail stuck in your finger (see Table 2). The painful stimulus travels along a pathway up the spinal column, which then activates the pain center in the brain. Typically, an injury always produces a painful experience that matches the injury, and there should be no pain without injury. In other words, it's an alert signal, like a fire alarm going off, telling us that something is wrong and to do something.

Table 2 shows a diagram of how pain is transmitted and registered.

Table 2

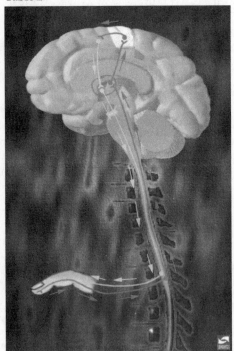

Chronic pain, however, where there is pain but no ongoing injury or in cases where pain stays around after an acute injury has healed, simply does not make sense. The fire alarm isn't needed any longer because we're alert, but we can't turn it off. To further explain this, research has shown that pain signals are sent to the brain through many routes. **Functional magnetic resonance imaging (fMRI)** studies have demonstrated that the experience of pain is actually recorded in many different areas of the brain simultaneously.

As discussed in earlier chapters, pain is based not just on a physical event, but also on your responses to the physical event: thoughts, emotions, and behaviors, which are affected by your gender, race, religion, social status, age, and so forth. It is the emotional experience of pain that has been shown to be especially important to your perception of pain and, ultimately, your suffering.

The main area in the midbrain where you form and register emotions is the limbic system. The limbic system is a set of brain structures that surround the thalamus (the pain-processing center) and is responsible for filtering and prioritizing all the impulses your brain receives. The limbic system is a central core of structures below the cerebral cortex. These structures include the **hypothalamus, hippocampus, insula, basal ganglia,** and **amygdala.** In addition to emotions, the limbic system has much to do with memories.

- The hypothalamus is a tiny area in the brain concerned with **homeostasis,** which keeps things level and even. If something changes, the hypothalamus is charged with returning us to a set point, like a thermostat. It regulates your body temperature, pulse, blood pressure, aggressive feelings, breathing, hunger, and arousal in response to emotional situations, thirst, pleasure, anger, sexual satisfaction, and more. The hypothalamus is also partly responsible for your responses to pain.

- The amygdalae are two small clumps of nerve cells on each side of the thalamus at one end of the hippocampus. They are involved in sexual responses, anger, aggression, and fear. They are the alert center—the initial warning system for the rest of the nervous system.

- The hippocampus is made up of two "horns" that curve back from the amygdalae. It is important in changing short-term memories into long-term memories and recording and recalling memories.

- The basal ganglia are located deep within the cerebral hemispheres in the back of the brain and are responsible for how you acquire and process knowledge, the coordination of movement, and voluntary movement.

- The insular cortex, also known as the insula, is part of the cerebral cortex. It is involved in virtually every human emotion and behavior. The insula controls perception, motor control, self-awareness, cognitive functioning, and interpersonal experience. It is also the part of the brain that judges the degree and significance of pain.

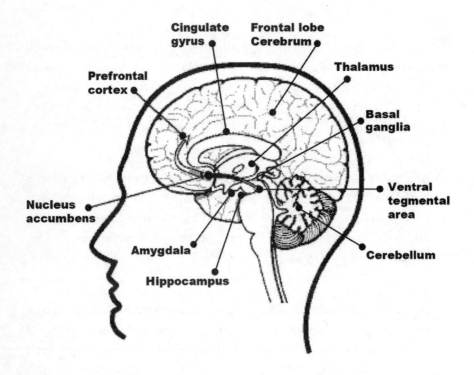

This simple diagram represents general areas of the brain.

The limbic system operates by influencing the **endocrine** (hormone) **system** and the **autonomic nervous system**. It is linked to smell, learning, memory, thinking, and sexual function, and helps you integrate functions connected to personal experiences. The limbic system is interconnected with the **nucleus accumbens**, the brain's "pleasure" or "reward" center. The nucleus accumbens plays a role in sexual arousal, as well as in getting high from certain drugs.

Other areas of the brain that function in concert with the limbic system include:

- The **cingulate gyrus,** which provides a path from the thalamus to the hippocampus and is believed to be responsible for focusing attention on emotionally significant events and for associating memories with smells and pain.

- The **ventral tegmental area** of the brain stem, consisting of pathways that are responsible for pleasure and reward.

- The **prefrontal cortex,** involved in planning for the future and taking action. It also appears to be involved in the same pathways as the ventral tegmental area and plays a role in addiction reward and pleasure.

- The **somatosensory cortex,** which processes input from the various systems in the body that are sensitive to touch. There are a number of different sensory experiences involved in touch, including specific sensitivity to pain and sensitivity to temperature. The somatosensory cortex is extremely sensitive, allowing people to detect and interpret a wide variety of sensations.

The autonomic nervous system plays an important role in emotions, and therefore has an impact on your experience of pain. It is made up of two parts, the **sympathetic nervous system** and the **parasympathetic nervous system.** These two systems function in opposition to each other. When they are in balance, homeostasis is achieved and the brain is balanced—you feel awake and comfortable.

The sympathetic nervous system prepares you for the kinds of activities associated with running from danger or preparing to fight it. It makes your heart pound, stimulates sweat glands, opens the bronchial tubes of the lungs, opens the eyes, and dilates the pupils (called the "fight-or-flight" response). This system also accepts information concerning pain in the internal organs. Because the nerves that carry information about organ pain also carry information about pain from other areas of the body, the information occasionally gets confused. This is the basis for

referred pain. A good example of referred pain is when someone feels pain in their jaw or arm when they're having a heart attack.

Nerve cells communicate by the transmission of certain chemicals called neurotransmitters. Neurotransmitters are involved with the experience of pain and all emotions. These chemicals are responsible for sending between nerves information about the pain and/or emotions being sensed. Many different types of nociceptors and brain centers receive this information and cause a variety of phenomena in the body. Neurotransmitters are classified based on whatever stimulus or stimuli they react to.

Some examples of a few neurotransmitters (there are hundreds of different neurotransmitters) and what they affect include:

- **Epinephrine** (adrenalin)—increases heart rate, contracts blood vessels, dilates air passages; also involved with the fight-or-flight response governed by the sympathetic nervous system.

- **Norepinephrine** (noradrenalin)—wakefulness, anxiety, alertness; also involved in pain.

- **Dopamine**—associated with addiction, love, basic rewards, drives for pleasure, and voluntary movement.

- **Acetylcholine**—voluntary movement and the regulation of smooth muscle and cardiac muscle. In the central nervous system, acetylcholine is involved in learning, memory, and mood.

- **GABA (gamma-aminobutyric acid)**—turnoff of motor neurons, resulting in relaxation and sleepiness.

- **Serotonin**—memory, emotions, mood, appetite, wakefulness, sleep, and temperature regulation. Serotonin also decreases pain.

During his years of chronic pain, Paul's limbic system was on tilt. Fear, anger, and frustration all became pain. This was because his dopamine, serotonin, and GABA levels were at low levels. His levels of epinephrine and norepinephrine were chronically elevated, causing him to feel anxiety, heart palpitations, more fear, and general uneasiness. He couldn't sleep, his appetite was off, and he was extremely irritable—all because of imbalances in his central nervous system.

His parasympathetic nervous system was underactive. The parasympathetic nervous system's job is to return the body to its normal state after an emergency. Among other things, it decreases heart rate, constricts the bronchial tubes, constricts the pupils, and calms you down. Paul couldn't seem to settle down and relax. His anxiety was running rampant, and there seemed to be nothing he could do about it except drink or take other drugs, which offered temporary relief.

From brain research, scientists have learned that specific pain centers exist that have evolved from the areas of the brain that control the body. According to one study, the overlap between these areas and emotion-processing regions of the brain explains the subjective qualities of human pain.

Jodie Anne Trafton, Ph.D., director of the Veterans Administration Palo Alto Health Care Systems Program Evaluation and Resource Center in California, further explains that pain is part of an **interoceptive** (or "well-being") **system** that tells you how you're feeling. This system, which involves the highly specialized areas of the brain I just described, is programmed differently from your other senses and is linked to the limbic and autonomic nervous systems. In addition to giving you a sense of yourself, the well-being system motivates you into action to correct internal states. In other words, it adjusts most of your functions, behaviors, internal "climate" (for example, blood pressure, heart rate, stomach acid), and emotions. It organizes and processes all the input and judges the importance of each of these internal states depending on the results—you sit down, yawn, go to the fridge, doze off, or become anxious. All these actions are attempts to return the organism (you) to a balanced state.

Dr. Trafton has been one of my best teachers about chronic pain. She describes research using functional magnetic resonance imaging (fMRI), which has shown that the area of the brain that controls the well-being system is activated by heat, exercise, anger, seeing emotions on the faces of others, and, most importantly, chronic pain. Basically, what this means is that you have an extremely complicated and complex system in your body that processes information about how you're doing in the world. The incoming information becomes your feelings, and you respond with drives.

"As pain becomes chronic, the sensory components become less important and the emotional and behavioral components tend to take on more importance," Trafton says. "It is because of learning. Having pain is a strong emotional experience. It will reshape your behavior. It will reshape how you interact with the world. And that in itself means your brain is going to respond differently over time."

In fact, researchers now know that when the brain responds differently, it actually changes physically and *becomes* different. Emotion and pain have caused the brain to change.

The Plastic Brain

The human brain is "plastic"—it can change both physically and functionally. Every day, the brain adapts and compensates in response to stimuli. Connections can be rewired and/or refined; the brain's gray matter can thicken, and new neurons or connections can be produced.

In the not-too-distant past, most scientists believed the brain was "hard-wired" and unchanging. Certain areas of the brain handled only certain functions. The accepted theory, for example, was that at birth, one portion of the human brain was wired to allow you to learn language and to speak, another area was wired for sight, and another area was wired to help you walk. Once you lost any given ability, that portion of the brain was also lost to you.

Recent research, however, has revealed that just the opposite is true. While you may lose the ability to walk because of a spinal injury, you don't lose the use of the part of the brain that helped you walk. The brain can adapt and change. For instance, without any conscious help from you, your brain can eventually begin using the walking area of the brain in some other way, for some other function. This is an example of brain plasticity, or **neuroplasticity**.

Neuroplasticity is an important part of your responses to many things, especially chronic pain. You change your ideas and perceptions in response to learning new things, and you experience new ideas and situations every day. That your brain actually undergoes physical changes as you learn or experience these new things may be a little harder to see, but this is also something that happens daily. Your plastic brain changes every time you learn a new word, try a new activity, encounter a new face, or experience a new pain.

Neuroplasticity is a physical process. Your gray matter can thicken or shrivel, and new wires can connect or disconnect. Research has shown that as your abilities shift, there is a direct link to the growth or reduction in the physical brain and in the number and types of connections each neuron makes.

Basically, what scientists have learned is that the brain can be physically changed when a person experiences chronic pain. For example, when you burn yourself, it hurts, and you feel it in an area of your brain. When the burn heals, the pain goes away and the brain is relieved, even happy. You go on as before. However, if the pain doesn't go away and continues to hurt, not only does your brain not return to normal, it changes physically. It becomes a different brain. FMRI studies have shown that certain areas of the brain decrease function with long-standing chronic pain.

The brain tends to decline with age. As you get older your memory slips, you don't hear or see as well, and learning new things isn't quite as easy. However, there are steps you can take that will help you use your brain's plasticity to full advantage. You can design the right therapy or exercise, and practice regularly.

As scientists learn more about the brain and its ability to change, the possibilities for treatments and applications of this knowledge become enormous. Research has proven that you can make changes in your brain just by thinking. A musician can make actual, physical changes in her brain merely by thinking about playing her instrument. By treating urges and compulsions as wayward brain chemistry, patients with **obsessive-compulsive disorder (OCD)** have changed the area of their brain that generates the OCD behavior. It has been demonstrated by people at risk of depression that by concentrated effort they can change their brain chemistry, thereby reducing their risk of depression.

It is clear that with chronic use of opioid medications and sedating substances, the brain changes and functions in a diminished capacity. Scans of the brain show a change in the level of dopamine transporters in the brains of such people. The net effects of these brain changes are decreased concentration, depressed mood, irritability, and problems with memory. Similarly, when drugs are eliminated from the brain, over time changes in the brain can be seen that parallel the behavioral improvements as recovery evolves.

As more and more is learned about neuroplasticity, scientists are creating more and more therapies and exercises designed to enhance brain functions. You simply have to use the right exercise(s) to change the brain in the most advantageous way. Studies have shown that by altering their behaviors using learned procedures, people can physically change their brains and the way they feel pain.

When Paul ran out of the opioids that had been so much a part of his life for so long, he found that at times he felt like he was going insane. He couldn't sleep; he had severe muscle spasms and was irritable beyond belief. He snapped at Lila for the least little thing. These actions were a reflection of his changed brain and his hyperactive sympathetic nervous system. Acutely, he was withdrawing from the physically dependence-inducing opioids (I will discuss this in more detail in Chapter Four).

As you will see in later chapters, when Paul finally gave up the opioids for good, though he wasn't consciously aware of it, his dopamine levels gradually returned to normal levels and his adrenaline levels decreased. His life started to improve because his brain was changing in positive ways. For now, this was not the case for him or Phyllis.

Phyllis became less and less functional. The more she hurt, the less she moved. She would go to bed and not get up for days at a time, much like her mother had done. Since she didn't move her muscles, they atrophied and she became thin all over, particularly in her arms and legs. She was drinking a lot of vodka by that time, so her liver swelled and her abdomen became distended. Her brain circuits started to shrivel up, her dopamine and serotonin levels bottomed out, and she became fatigued and despondent.

Both Paul and Phyllis reflect the phenomenon we have just discussed. Both took significant amounts of medication to their detriment, though that is not the case for all people who take medications. Phyllis and Paul became addicted and out of control. Opioid painkillers will be discussed in much greater detail in the next chapter.

CHAPTER 4

Falling Down the Rabbit Hole

Opioids and Chronic Pain

"The aim of the wise is not to secure pleasure,
but to avoid pain."

Aristotle

Pain is the most frequent reason Americans seek medical attention, and its treatment is the specialty of thousands of professionals across the United States. Unfortunately, pain is most often inadequately treated, which leads to enormous social costs.

By far, the most prevalent treatments for pain are medications. They are the easiest method of treating pain, requiring the least amount of effort by physicians and patients. They work quickly and provide relief (at least, at first). In our culture, physicians are encouraged to treat chronic pain in order to spare the patients suffering. Pain is the "fifth vital sign" and should be measured and treated. Perceived barriers to "proper" prescribing of opioids are to be overcome. Those doctors who are reluctant to prescribe them are labeled "opiophobic." In this decade, there has been a proliferation of pain clinics notorious for overprescribing large amounts of painkillers without proper evaluation and follow-up. Impediments to the use of opioids include concerns about addiction, side effects, tolerance, and possible problems with regulatory agencies for overprescribing.

For years the number of people experiencing chronic pain and coexisting psychological disorders including addiction has been increasing significantly. In 2003, according to Peter D. Hart Research Associates, the majority of adults in the United States (57 percent) have experienced chronic or recurrent pain in the last year. According to the American Chronic Pain Association, there are approximately 100 million Americans suffering from chronic pain.

Research published in *Pain Physician Journal* (2006) reports that 90 percent of people in the United States receiving treatment for pain management are prescribed opiate medication. Of that number, 18 percent to 41 percent had opiate abuse/addiction problems. At least eighty billion dollars is spent for pain relief in the United States each year, a significant amount of which is for prescription medications. What is harder to quantify is the emotional cost to family systems when one or more members suffer with a chronic pain condition.

According to some professionals, we have entered an era of a prescription drug epidemic. Deaths related to overdose of opioids are on the rise, and since 2006 opioids have become the number-one most abused legal drug in the United States. Because of this, the DEA and FDA have created a panel of experts to develop Risk Evaluation and Mitigation Strategies (REMS) to minimize the risk of inappropriate prescribing and bad outcomes.

Medications for Pain

There are two groups of medications used to treat pain, **adjuvants** and **analgesics**. Adjuvants are medications that have primary uses other than pain relief, but often are helpful in relieving pain. They include antidepressants, muscle relaxants, and anticonvulsants.

Analgesics are drugs specifically used in treating pain. They include opioids, nonopioids, and combination medications that have both opioid and nonopioid ingredients. The World Health Organization recommends starting pain treatment with nonopioid over-the-counter medications such as aspirin, acetaminophen (Tylenol), and others. Nonsteroidal anti-inflammatory drugs (**NSAID**s) are commonly prescribed and also are available as over-the-counter and prescription pain medications. Since inflammation often adds to many types of pain, NSAIDs are especially useful. They include aspirin, ibuprofen (Advil, Motrin), naproxen (Naprosyn), anaprox (Aleve), indomethacin (Indocin), nabumetone (Relafen), and others. The NSAIDs work to block prostaglandin, a chemical that produces pain at the site of injury or inflammation. Celecoxib (Celebrex) is in a class of anti-inflammatory drugs called COX-2 inhibitors, which work similarly to traditional NSAIDs but are easier on the stomach. Steroids such as prednisone are very potent anti-inflammatory medications and are used in some types of painful conditions. In addition to the drugs listed below, there are topical formulations of a number of medications. Some are packaged as lidocaine patches (Lidoderm), diclofenac patches (Flector), capsaicin (Zostrix), and diclofenac gel (Voltaren). Nonopioid medications, including analgesics and adjuvants, are listed in Table 3.

Opioids and combination drugs are the most-prescribed medications available today for those in chronic pain.

Opioids and combination drugs are the most-prescribed medications available today for those in chronic pain. They have extremely effective analgesic or pain-relieving properties. They are the most powerful pain-relieving drugs and are the foundation in the treatment of severe acute and chronic pain. These drugs offer relief from chronic pain, and the use of opioids is on the rise. From 1997 to 2005, major opioid sales rose 90 percent, with over 200,000 pounds purchased. That's 300 milligrams of opioids to every American! The cost of drug marketing in 1997 was $11 billion; by 2005 that number had reached $30 billion. Those figures alone are quite sobering.

Medications that fall into the opioid class (see Table 4), in order of decreasing strength, include fentanyl (Actiq, Duragesic), morphine (Avinza, Kadian, MS Contin), methadone, meperidine (Demerol), hydromorphone (Dilaudid), buprenorphine (Subutex, Suboxone, Butrans), oxycodone (Oxycontin, Oxyfast, Percodan, Tylox), hydrocodone (Lorcet, Norco), codeine (Tylenol with Codeine), and

Table 3

Non-Opioid Medications		
Drug Class		**Generic**	**Brand Name(s)**

Drug Class		Generic	Brand Name(s)
Anticonvulsants		Gabapentin	Neurontin
		Topiramate	Topamax
		Carbemazepine	Tegretol
		Valproic Acid	Depakote
		Pregablin	Lyrica
Anti-depressants	*Tricyclics*	Amitryptilline	Elavil
		Desipramine	Norpramin
		Norpramine	Pamelor
	SSRI–SNRI	Venflaxine	Effexor
		Duloxetine	Cymbalta
NSAIDs	*COX 2s Traditional NSAIDs*	Celecoxib	Celebrex
		Ibuprofen	Advil, Motrin
		Naproxen	Naprosyn, Aleve
		Indomethacin	Indocin
		Nabunetone	Relafen
Muscle Relaxants		Methocarbamol	Robaxin
		Liorisal	Baclofen
		Metaxalone	Skelaxin
		Cyclobenzaprine	Flexeril
		Tizanadine	Xanaflex
Topicals		Capascins	Zostrix
		Lidocaine	Lidoderm patches
		Diclofenac gel	Voltaren
		Diclofenac patches	Flector

propoxyphene (Darvon and Darvocet, which were recently removed from the market). Combination drugs include Lortab and Vicodin, both of which contain hydrocodone and acetaminophen; Percocet, which contains acetaminophen and oxycodone; and Darvocet and Tylenol 3 and 4, which contain acetaminophen and propoxyphene or codeine, respectively. Tramadol (Ultram, Ultracet) is not chemically

Table 4

Mood-altering & Potentially Addictive Drugs
(This list is not all-inclusive.)

Type	Brand Name	Generic Name
Amphetamines	Adderall	Amphetamine aspartate/Sulfate
	Dexedrine	Dextroamphetamine
Barbiturates	Fioricet/Codeine	Butalbital/Codeine/Acet/Caffeine
	Fiorinal	Butalbital/Aspirin/Caffeine
	Phenobarbital	Phenobarbital
Benzodiazepines	Ativan	Lorazepam
	Dalmane	Flurazepam
	Halcion	Triazolam
	Klonopin	Clonazepam
	Librium	Chlordiazepoxide
	Restoril	Temazepam
	Serax	Oxazepam
	Tranxene	Clorazepate Dipotassium
	Valium	Diazepam
	Xanax	Alprazolam
Hypnotics (for sleep)	Ambien	Zolpidem titrate
	Lunesta	Eszopiclone
	Sonata	Zaleplon
Muscle Relaxants	Soma	Carisoprodol
	Equagesic	Meprobamate/Aspirin
Opioids	Hycodan	Hydrocodone/Methylbromide
	Tussionex	Hydrocodone bit/Chlorpheneramine
	Actiq	Oral transmucosal fentanyl citrate
	Avinza	Morphine sulfate
	Demerol	Meperidine
	Dilaudid	Hydromorphone
	Duragesic	Fentanyl
	Kadian	Morphine sulfate
	Methadone	Methadone
	MS Contin	Morphine sulfate
	Oxycontin	Oxycodone
	Oxyfast	Oxycodone
	Percocet	Oxycodone/Acetaminophen
	Percodan	Oxycodone/Aspirin
	Tylox	Oxycodone/Acetaminophen

continued on page 46

Table 4 (continued)

Mood-altering & Potentially Addictive Drugs Continued *(This list is not all-inclusive.)*		
Type	**Brand Name**	**Generic Name**
Opioids	Lorcet	Hydrocodone/Acetaminophen
	Lortab	Hydrocodone/Acetaminophen
	Norco	Hydrocodone/Acetaminophen
	Subutex	Buprenorphine hydrochloride
	Suboxone	Buprenorphine hydrochloride + naloxone
	Tylenol/Codeine	Acetaminophen/Codeine
	Vicodin	Hydrocodone/Acetaminophen
	Vicoprofen	Hydrocodone/Ibuprofen
	Darvocet-N	Propoxyphene/Acetaminophen
	Darvon	Propoxyphene
	Stadol NS	Butorphanol tartrate
	Talwin NX	Pentazocine naloxone
Stimulants	Concerta	Methylphenidate
	Ritalin	Methylphenidate

an opioid; however, it works by the same mechanism as opioids and can cause similar effects and problems. The American Academy of Pain Medicine, the American Pain Society, and the World Health Organization have endorsed opioids, also called narcotic analgesics, where necessary, as an essential part of a pain management plan.

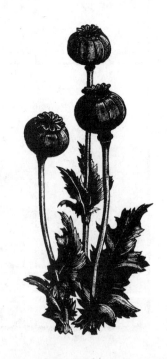

Opioids were originally derived from opium, a bitter, grainy powder that comes from the seedpod of the poppy flower. Today, most of the opioid analgesics are made synthetically. Opium has been used for millennia as a pain reliever. Fossil remains of poppy-seed cakes and poppy pods were discovered in 4,000-year-old Swiss dwellings. During America's first centuries, pilgrims grew poppies and then mixed them with whisky to ease aches and pains.

In the early nineteenth century, morphine was isolated from opium, and it quickly became a primary ingredient in many medicines to treat pain, diarrhea, and colic in infants. Mothers and babysitters found that opium-based concoctions kept their kids happy and docile. They were sold under such names as Ayer's Cherry Pectoral, Mrs. Winslow's Soothing Syrup, Darby's Carminative, Paregoric Elixir, and McMunn's Elixir of Opium. Some were teething syrups for young children, some were "soothing syrups," some were recommended for diarrhea and dysentery, and some were used

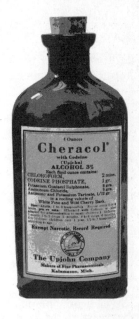

for "women's trouble." These formulations were advertised in newspapers and magazines and on billboards as "painkillers," "women's friends," and "consumption cures." It has been reported that during this heyday of opium, one wholesale drug house distributed more than 600 proprietary medicines and other products containing opiates.

Tincture of opium, known as laudanum, was a common product used in the Victorian era to ease mild pain and relieve boredom. It was viewed as a medicine and not a drug of abuse, such as heroin or "chloral," the popular name for chloral hydrate. Sigmund Freud believed that the use of cocaine was a cure for morphine and alcohol addiction, as well as a remedy for all sorts of ailments. He also learned of the intense habit-forming nature of cocaine through this failed clinical experiment. However, along with opium's enthusiastic popularity came its tragic downside: It is estimated that in 1839, opium and its preparations were responsible for more premature deaths than any other chemical agent.

By the 1940s, opioids were tightly controlled and could be obtained and used only if they were prescribed by physicians. Laws became so strict that doctors could lose their licenses if they inappropriately prescribed opioids. As a result, because of legal fears, doctors became reluctant to prescribe opioids, and pain was vastly undertreated.

During the second half of the twentieth century, pain-treatment advocates and pharmaceutical companies helped reestablish opioid treatment for pain due to cancer and other life-ending diseases. As a result, opioids have been readily used to help relieve chronic cancer pain because of the prevailing attitude that "if people with cancer are dying anyway, we should make them comfortable without worrying about long-term effects like addiction." Even more recently, a growing number of physicians began prescribing opioids as therapy for chronic noncancer pain as well.

Managing Pain

Reasonable goals of pain management are to reduce discomfort by 50 percent or more without impairing function, and, where possible, improving function. It is clear that long-term opioid treatment for people with chronic pain is quite appropriate for some. The best way to tell if the opioids are working for you is to answer three questions:

1   Is your pain totally or mostly relieved, or at least
    significantly better?

2   Is your function maintained or improved?

3   Are the side effects (constipation, fatigue, mental clouding,
    itching, nausea, vomiting, urinary problems, constricted pupils,
    dizziness, sweating, muscle and bone pain, confusion, muscle
    spasms, and sedation) absent or tolerable?

If the answer to these questions is yes, then you can stop reading this chapter now. This is successful opioid treatment and needs no intervention.

After Paul's spinal surgery, he found himself consumed with the pain. His life had become unbearable. He could not sleep, take a deep breath, walk, stand, or do any of the things most people take for granted without discomfort.

Although Paul had been taking pain medications for months after his last surgery, they weren't quelling the pain. With urging and occasional demands by Paul, his doctors prescribed stronger and stronger opioids. It wasn't long before he was in a prescription program that included an extremely strong time-release opioid (morphine SR, slow-release), as well as a short-acting drug (Lortab) for breakthrough pain. He was also taking zolpidem (Ambien) to sleep and carisoprodol (Soma) as a muscle relaxant. The medications were not the perfect answer, but they worked to get rid of the pain, sort of.

One of the main tenets of opioid therapy is that the dosage should be set at a level at which pain is controlled with the least amount of side effects. Unfortunately for Paul, he soon began to experience many of the unwanted side effects of these potent drugs. His pain was numbed, but so were his mind, his speech, and his emotions. There were times when he would sit in a stupor in his bedroom, unable to communicate. His mind was not as sharp. His memory was foggy. The drugs Paul took to control the pain had begun to smother his life. He could not work or even carry out many functions around the house.

Meet Sam

Sam had suffered with chronic pain for as long as he could remember. When he was fifteen, his scoliosis got the better of him and he went for a surgical evaluation. He had worn a brace for years before that and had steeled himself to the taunts and name-calling. Sometimes he felt like he really was the "hunchback," which is what the other kids called him. Sam was brought up by loving and supportive, though clueless, parents who did the best they could, which wasn't nearly enough. As far as he was concerned he was damaged goods, and his responses were bitterness, frustration, anger, resentment, and depression. By the time he turned fourteen, he had started doing his own investigations about the condition that plagued him and started lobbying for surgery, which looked like it would happen in his sixteenth year. He could barely contain himself at the thought that his hump would be gone and he would be free of pain for the first time in his life.

Either he wasn't told the truth or he couldn't hear it from the doctor, but either way, he was totally optimistic with unbridled enthusiasm as the day of his surgery approached. He'd never taken anything stronger than Tylenol and wanted to keep it that way. He'd seen a schoolmate overdose and die from prescription painkillers, and he had no intention of getting hooked.

When he awoke from surgery, he couldn't believe the stabbing pain that ran up and down his spine. He felt like he imagined his favorite superhero in the X-Men series felt when he had been infused with metal. Over the next few weeks, snowed by powerful opioids and sedatives, he began to get used to the stiff feeling, and when he arose from bed he realized that his new position in space was upright—unbending, but straight up. He had gained four inches, and he felt like his hopes and prayers were answered. Weeks turned to months, and even with therapy his pain persisted as it had before, but the fact that his hump was gone made it all worth it.

By the time Sam was twenty-three, the fusion had seemed to lose its effectiveness. His pain increased, and his posture was exhaustingly stiff and unyielding. He became angrier, and was now irreversibly scarred by the deforming surgery. He added his team of doctors and nurses to his list of resentments, and he cursed the day he let himself be talked into having the crummy surgery. Before surgery he had pain, but nothing like what was developing now. All of his childhood demons were back with a vengeance. He felt unloving and unlovable.

Finally giving in to the urging of his mom, Eleanor, Sam consulted a pain doctor. He had struggled for over three years—not sleeping, losing weight, irritable all the time, and barely holding on at work, where he was a software analyst. He had alienated the few friends he had made, and spent his time playing video games. He had mastered most of them, but was miserable.

He left work early on a Tuesday and met Dr. Joe, who ordered an MRI and referred Sam immediately to a neurosurgeon who specialized in scoliosis. The surgeon was not terribly helpful, stating that he could redo the surgery, which would require a year-long recuperation period. Sam vetoed this, stating that he'd rather die than go though another torturing surgery. He returned to Dr. Joe for pain management.

The medications started slowly—hydrocodone four times per day, with gabapentin (Neurontin) for the tingling neuropathic pain he felt in his legs and feet. This gave him relief from his pain for the first time in years. He still couldn't sleep, so on the next visit Dr. Joe prescribed triazolam (Halcion), which was effective. Over the next few months the medications proved less effective, and Dr. Joe advanced the dosage and potency of the drugs from hydrocodone to oxycodone to morphine and finally to methadone. By the end of the year, Sam's pain was barely controlled by four to six methadone tablets per day. He needed two Halcion per night by then, and was so tired all the time that he ended up taking amphetamine (Adderal) to give him a little energy. His life not only didn't improve, it got worse. He was more irritable than ever, snapping at people in supermarkets and on the street, spiraling downward in the face of increasing frustration, anger, anxiety, and unrelenting depression.

The methadone barely lasted an hour and only blunted the pain, offering minimal relief. He tried to stop numerous times; however, the withdrawals were overwhelming as he experienced body aches, nausea, and anxiety that caused him to restart his pills. The longest he ever lasted was six hours without the drug. After a few years of this endless cycle of pain and pill taking, Sam became so sick and tired of living the only way he knew how to live that he decided to end it all. He lined up his pills one night and started taking them. It was the first time he ever took an amount in excess of his prescribed dosage. He woke up the next day in the intensive care unit. He later learned that he had been found by his mother, who showed up at his apartment when she was unable to reach him by phone.

How Do Opioids Work?

Opioids' effects are caused by activating receptors located throughout the brain and spinal cord. The two important effects of opioids are pain relief and enhanced mood. Once an opioid medication reaches these receptors, it activates the opioid receptors and produces an effect of relieving pain. It also causes mood enhancement in the form of stress reduction and euphoria, for some. The brain produces many natural endorphins that activate opioid receptors and relieve pain. As discussed in Chapter Three, these chemicals have been linked to many functions of the brain including pain relief, GI activities, respiration, mood, and hormonal regulation.

When you take an opioid, it encourages your brain to release greater amounts of dopamine, which causes a brief, intense sense of well-being, followed by a relaxed state. Opioids help ease pain by interfering with the pain messages traveling to your brain. Pleasure and relief from pain are closely connected in your brain.

Pleasure and relief from pain are closely connected in your brain.

Unfortunately, in addition to the desirable pain-relieving qualities of opioids, the drugs can have negative effects. Some of the side effects reported by those who take opioids include difficulty concentrating, blurred vision, reduced respiratory rate, nausea, vomiting, constipation, itching, sleepiness, insomnia, low energy, fatigue, anxiety, and depression. Another problem with opioid therapy, as with Paul and Sam, is that it is often combined with other habit-forming medications such as sedatives, alcohol, sleeping pills, and stimulants. The net effect is that many people are maintained on several long-term prescriptions, with significant consequences and no end in sight.

Many millions of people are being started and continued on opioids for chronic pain with no plan for stopping them in the future. According to Doug Gourlay, MD, Director of Pain and Chemical Dependency, Wasser Pain Management Centre, Mount Sinai Hospital, Toronto, Canada, and Howard Heit, MD, internist, gastroenterologist, and chronic pain specialist in Fairfax, Virginia, a management consideration when beginning opioid treatment should include an "exit strategy" for those in whom the opioids are not working or where side effects exceed benefits. Doctors should prescribe opioids where needed, but always with an eye to stopping them in the future, especially if they aren't successfully treating the chronic pain. Herb Malinoff, MD, often says, "Don't take off if you don't know how to land. Plan an exit strategy before starting these medications."

Physicians see large numbers of people who, though on large doses of opioid medications, continue to have significant levels of pain. Furthermore, they suffer because of the side effects of the medications. Even worse, they notice they're not doing the things they used to. They aren't playing with the kids, going out with friends and family, performing at work or school, and generally feeling well enough to participate in life. For some, the pain is the same or only slightly decreased after a dose of medication, and their function is worsened. Instead of being helped, many find themselves prisoners of these medications. Sam kept increasing the dose in an attempt to gain some pain relief, but he found the medications to be less and less effective. Sam had developed tolerance.

Tolerance, according to the Liaison Committee on Pain and Addiction (LCPA), is "a state of adaptation in which exposure to a drug induces changes that result in a diminution of one or more of the drug's effects over time," meaning it requires more of the medication to have the same effect as it did when the individual first started taking it. The person's body adapts to the presence of the drug and he or she needs more of it to feel the same amount of pain relief. This often can lead to more pill taking and less relief and comfort. One might increase the dose, and doctors might prescribe more potent medications to overcome the tolerance.

What is even worse for many people is that when they try to stop these medications, they can't. Many people who take opioids for longer than a month or two develop **physical dependence** and have some degree of **withdrawal** discomfort if they stop. Generally speaking, the longer a person takes the opioid and the higher the dose, the worse the withdrawal will be.

According to the Liaison Committee on Pain and Addiction of the American Academy of Pain Medicine, the American Pain Society, and the American Society of Addiction Medicine, "physical dependence is a state of adaptation that is manifested by a drug class-specific withdrawal syndrome that can be produced by abrupt cessation, rapid dose reduction, decreasing blood level of the drug, and/or administration of an **antagonist**." Dr. Gourlay and Dr. Heit point out that many different types of nonaddictive drugs, including corticosteroids, antidepressants, and others, can also cause dependence in a person. A person who is dependent on a drug will experience uncomfortable sensations if he or she abruptly stops taking it or decreases the dose. This is called withdrawal, which Sam experienced when he tried to stop his medications on numerous occasions. It is the avoidance of withdrawal that drives some people to continue taking these medications even when they want to stop them.

Withdrawal from Opioids

If you are dependent on opioids, sedatives, or tranquilizers (any medications listed in Table 3), withdrawal can start just hours after you have taken your last dose. You can experience restlessness, muscle and bone pain, insomnia, diarrhea, vomiting, and other symptoms. If you are going through withdrawal, you may require medical attention. Typically, major withdrawal symptoms hit their worst point within seventy-two hours and gradually subside over the course of the next five to seven days. These symptoms vary widely from person to person and with different drugs and different formulations of drugs.

Opioids also can produce what is sometimes described as **withdrawal-mediated pain**. The pain-relieving effect of some opioids lasts only a few hours, and then the pain returns even more intensely as these drugs wear off. Many who take opioids for long periods have intermittent withdrawal between doses, and hence increased pain.

Addiction is also a possibility with chronic use of opioids in some people. Another problem that makes it difficult to stop taking opioids for some is that they not only have an effect on the pain center of the brain, but they also affect the reward/pleasure center of the brain's limbic system. As discussed in Chapter Three, the limbic system is connected to and works in harmony with the nucleus accumbens, the brain's pleasure center. The nucleus accumbens plays a role in sexual arousal, appetite, and the "high" from certain drugs. The limbic system has been linked to smell, learning, memory, processing of cognitive data, and sexual function.

For some who take opioids, rather than feeling sleepy or woozy they get a burst of energy. They suddenly find the motivation to clean the house, wash the car, go shopping, or do any number of other chores. Some find they can only go to work if they take their medication. This is partly because the pain is lessened, but also because the drug is having an effect on other neurotransmitters in the limbic system, especially dopamine. As Dr. Barry Rosen said, "My patient took a Vicodin and her marriage got better." This means that some people take the medications for the stimulating effect and not just the relief of pain, as originally intended by the prescribing doctor. It is a particular problem for these people after they stop because they are left, for a time (weeks to several months), with a lowered energy level, which is part of **protracted withdrawal**. In an effort to relieve the incapacitating fatigue, many people are driven to start back on the drug to relieve these symptoms.

Phyllis, by age twenty-four, was hooked on opioids as well as other drugs. She had to take six Percocets in the morning to get started. The Percocet gave her energy but left her feeling edgy, so she frequently would take two or three Xanax if she had them. If she didn't have the Xanax, she would drink a few beers or smoke some marijuana to mellow her out. She would move through her day, decreasing her pain, which by then had been diagnosed as fibromyalgia. Her body ached and her life was a drag. Light touch caused excruciating pain. The only thing that offered any relief—though fleeting and temporary—was the handful of Percocet she took on a regular basis. Frustrated with her agony, Phyllis had now taken to chewing these pills in an effort to bring quicker relief. She also struggled with constipation, a common and miserable side effect of opioids. She had a bowel movement no more than once a week even though she consumed large amounts of laxatives.

She found that if she crushed and snorted Oxycontin, the slow-release form of oxycodone, she could get instant pain relief and get quite a "high." Her boyfriend and dealer also showed her how to smoke the crushed powder, and eventually she started injecting it. This landed her in the hospital with an overdose (in combination with cocaine and five to six Valiums [diazepam] she had taken that day). "At least I was out of pain for a while," she said the next week to her Aunt Ellie, who came to take care of her.

The complexity of effects of the opioids is that in addition to relieving physical pain, they also diminish emotional pain. As a result, you may find you are using these drugs as a "chemical coper," that is, you are taking your prescriptions because you feel anxious, irritable, fearful, or depressed and the drugs work to temporarily relieve these symptoms. As with many chemicals that alter mood, the effect you take the pill for is soon replaced by a worsening of the state you were in before you took the pill.

It is common to take pain medication to relieve the depression associated with or caused by unremitting chronic pain. Recent studies reveal that the rate of major depression is directly related to the amount of pain a person feels; the greater the pain, the more likely there also will be symptoms of depression. In a study done at Stanford University, researchers showed that compared with those who have no symptoms of depression, those with major depression are more than twice as likely to have a chronic, painful condition.

In addition to tolerance and physical dependence, another potential downside to opioids is a condition called **opioid-induced hyperalgesia**.

Hyperalgesia means more pain. Opioids can also cause changes in the nervous system that can heighten your perception of pain and make you have more pain and feel worse. Jianren Mao, MD, Ph.D., Director for Translational Pain Research at Massachusetts General Hospital in Boston, and Jane Balantyne, MD, FRCA, Associate Professor of Anesthesia, Harvard Medical School, have found that long-term opioid use in some individuals is associated with this abnormal sensitivity to pain. This condition has been seen in many people with chronic pain who have been on long-term opioid therapy. In other words, for some who take opioids, the medication is actually making the pain worse. The solution to this condition is to decrease or, preferably, discontinue the opioids. This, of course, must be done under medical supervision. Studies have shown that many people have less pain after opioids are stopped. That certainly has been the case in my clinical practice.

> ### *Studies have shown that many people have less pain after opioids are stopped.*

Furthermore, it has been shown that opioids have an impact on the immune system. Scientists report that long-term exposure to opioids has a greater effect than short-term use, and abrupt withdrawal may also cause immune system problems. While researchers know all opioids have an impact on the immune system, some, such as morphine and heroin, have been shown to be worse, especially in people who have HIV/AIDS. Opioids also affect the sleep cycle, and in some cases cause periods of apnea. Sexual function and desire may be affected by opioid use and withdrawal, with decreased performance and changing levels of sex hormones, e.g., testosterone, prolactin, and/or estrogen.

Many people find that what started out as a positive influence and sensible antidote to pain actually makes the pain and suffering worse and causes increasing problems with health. It would make sense to simply stop the medications when this happens, but it's easier said than done. Giving up these medications often seems like being asked to give up a good friend and the only thing that appears to work to dampen the pain.

This is not to say that all prescription medications are bad or that they should be put aside in all cases. It is to say that if your medications are making you feel worse, you may benefit from a frank discussion with your prescribing doctor about the pros and cons of continuing or stopping your medications.

If you decide to stop your medications, even after the acute withdrawal phase, which may last a week or two, your energy level may not be normal for a while. It would not be uncommon for you to feel **dysphoric**, or kind of "off your game"—irritable, low-energy, with a depressed mood. It is possible not only to slow the progressively increasing doses of opioids, but to stop them all together.

Abruptly stopping your medication is not something you should do. For anyone who has taken opioids for any length of time, slow weaning or medically managed withdrawal is the safest way to get off pain drugs. It makes the most sense to get some professional help.

For many, heavy withdrawal lasts three or four days, and for Sam it took six weeks before all the withdrawal symptoms subsided. But it's important to know that the symptoms *will subside*.

Phyllis and Paul continued to struggle with chronic pain; the doses escalated and became more complicated. Her life spiraled downward into the syndrome known as addiction.

Important Information about Discontinuing Medications

Caution: *Do not* simply stop your medications. Over time, your body may have become accustomed to them and may be physically dependent on them. You must consult a knowledgeable health care provider or treatment center to supervise withdrawal from habit-forming medications including opioids, sedatives, hypnotics, and alcohol. Stopping these medications suddenly may be dangerous.

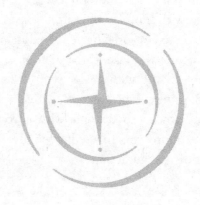

CHAPTER 5

Drug Addiction

"My head had my body convinced that I had pain and
needed to take pills to relieve the pain."

Ken Butler

Addiction is a chronic brain disease that affects millions in the United States. Despite harmful, often fatal consequences, people with the disease of addiction habitually and compulsively seek and use both legal and illegal drugs. Each person's vulnerability to addiction is different, but it has been proven that for some, once they begin using drugs, the structure of their brain and the way it works changes. These changes have profound effects that can last for the lifetime of the person using the drug.

For some, chronic pain and addiction go hand in hand. It's an unfortunate link, because addiction complicates the course of chronic pain in some who take opioids for pain relief. Many professionals believe the number of people who can be helped through opioid treatment far outnumbers those with the risk of addiction. However, some who stay on these medications do develop addiction. Further, those with a history of addiction who develop chronic pain are more likely to have problems if they take opioid painkillers. In order to more fully understand the relationship between addiction and chronic pain, it is necessary first to discuss exactly what addiction is.

For decades, professionals engaged in heated arguments about whether addiction is truly a disease or merely a behavior the addict could control if he or she really wanted to. While research increasingly confirms that using drugs changes the brains of addicts, those who believe addiction is a behavioral disorder and not a disease insist that before addiction reared its ugly head in a person's life, that person exercised his or her free will by *choosing* to use or not to use drugs. Behavior theorists and concerned family members further argue that even after a person is an active addict, there is nothing forcing that person to continue taking drugs: "He could stop if he really wanted to, if he used will power," or "She could stop if she cared enough about me." They claim those who have "real" diseases, such as diabetes or heart disease, have no say in the manifestation of their afflictions.

This view of addiction is simply wrong. One client asked me, "What's the difference between addiction and just really, *really* liking the drug?"

According to Dr. Alan I. Leshner, former director of the National Institute on Drug Abuse (NIDA), addiction unequivocally is a brain disease. We know exactly which parts of the brain are affected by addiction, and, in fact, a person doesn't necessarily even have to use drugs to have a predilection for addiction. The argument that addiction is substantially different from other diseases such as diabetes and heart disease, and that addicts only become addicts when they start to use drugs, isn't correct.

I'll use heart disease as an example: You are born with particularly narrow arteries in your heart and you have a tendency to produce too much cholesterol. You exercise faithfully your entire life, never eat fatty food, and stay away from red meat, sugar, and other foods that can contribute to heart disease, thereby staying healthy. Then you live a full life and die from natural causes before your system can produce enough plaque to clog your narrow heart arteries. That you didn't manifest the symptoms of heart disease doesn't mean you didn't have it, but rather that it didn't show up. On the other hand, if you smoke cigarettes, don't exercise, and eat foods full of saturated fat, would you be blamed for the ensuing heart attack that developed? Do you think it is the same as someone with a predisposition to becoming addicted who overused alcohol and developed cirrhosis of the liver? Drinking in that case would be like eating fatty foods and smoking—not a great idea, but not clearly pathological until it is too late. Addiction *seems* different.

Behavior is a symptom of addiction.

Addiction is a stigmatized disease, since most of the symptoms of addiction are behavioral. It appears that these behaviors are volitional. People who are addicted often do bad things—they affect those of us who love and care about them. They lie, cheat, steal, and hurt us. Because of this sense that these negative behaviors are under the addict's control, society tends to blame and judge the addict. I can assure you that an addict's actions are no more volitional than controlling blood pressure, sugar level, or a bad case of diarrhea with the flu. *Behavior is a symptom of addiction.* This does not mean that addicts are not responsible for their behavior or the damage it causes. They certainly need to face the consequences of what they have done, but they need help, as does any sick person. Addicts must get help first to stop the drug use, and then they can begin to work on the behaviors, examine their thoughts and feelings, and repair the damage they've caused.

What Makes Addicts Different?

The brains of addicts are wired differently from those of nonaddicts, and the disease of addiction is present in many brains well before a drug is ever used. Not everyone who is predisposed to addiction becomes an addict. On the other hand, there are people who develop the need to take higher or more frequent doses after trying a drug for a short period of time. A team of American researchers at Brown University in Rhode Island showed that even a single dose of morphine physically changed the brain, and the change persisted long after the effects of the drug had worn off. Other studies have shown that a single dose of methamphetamine has resulted in brain damage.

The parts of the brain that are abnormal in addicts are located in the limbic system—the midbrain where drives to survive emanate from. As discussed previously, this is also the area of the brain where emotions are perceived, pleasure is experienced, and physical and emotional pain occurs. It appears that the fundamental difference in the brains of addicts is *the way the drugs work* in their brains. This is the enhanced effect of dopamine release: increased pleasure, resulting in the development of an ongoing desire to use the drug.

People who are addicted to drugs may have made a decision at one time to try a drug, but they never made a decision to become addicts. Research has shown that the addict's brain was different before the first use of a drug; however, all the significant ways the brain changes in response to exposure to drugs are still being discovered. According to Dr. Leshner, "the evidence suggests that those long-lasting brain changes are responsible for the distortions of cognitive and emotional functioning that characterize addicts, particularly including the compulsion to use drugs that is the essence of addiction."

Addiction is more than a pharmacologic phenomenon related to a person's using enough drugs to cause tolerance and physical dependence. Currently, addiction is defined as a chronic, relapsing brain disease characterized by compulsive drug seeking and use, despite harmful consequences. In fact, a person could have addiction without developing tolerance or dependence. Addiction is best diagnosed by observing drug-using behavior over a period of time—until then, it can be concluded that there is "problematic use," which may end up evolving into addiction.

Drug dependence (a synonym for addiction) is really a syndrome of behaviors involving continued problematic use of mood-altering substances over a period of a year or more. Symptoms involve problems with controlling use, thus having an unpredictable outcome once a person begins using a substance. Furthermore, addicts often try to cut down or stop, but are unable to "stay stopped." They are preoccupied with the drug and keep using it even though it causes problems for them and those who care about them. People with addiction tend to stop doing the things they used to and "chase the high." In other words, they spend their time and energy looking for the drug, getting the drug, using the drug even though it is ruining their lives, and recovering from the effects of the drug when they stop using.

Eventually the addict becomes hooked physically and psychologically. Addiction is also a spiritual disease, in essence robbing the person of his or her spirit and soul. Addicts develop cravings for their drug of choice when it is absent from their systems, and they want to use it again and again. When they stop, they can experience unpleasant physical and psychological reactions. When the drug has been gone for a while, the addict craves the drug once again, which in many cases causes **relapse**—a return to using.

Brain imaging studies reported by NIDA show that addicted individuals have physical changes in areas of the brain critical to judgment, decision-making, learning, memory, and behavior control. It is believed these changes alter the way the brain works and may help explain the compulsive and destructive behaviors of addiction. Every drug leaves its own signature on the brain, and while all of the different drugs of abuse share a similar way of affecting the brain's reward center, each drug also has a unique way of changing how the brain functions. These changes include altering memory processes and thinking; changing motor skills, such as walking and talking; and causing extreme mood changes, such as depression, anxiety, fearfulness, aggression, and paranoia. In many instances, the drug can become the single most powerful motivator in an addict's existence. Once addicted, he or she will do almost anything to get more of the drug. The drug hijacks the reward center and becomes the primary drive. In other words, as Phyllis finally admitted, "I *need* the drug more than food, relationships, sleep, or personal safety. I need the drug to survive." It is a consequence of the hijacked brain overriding the thoughtful, moral, rational frontal lobe functions of the individual. The addict loses the ability to exert executive decision-making, being driven instead by more instinctive drives co-opted by the drugs.

Factors Influencing Addiction

As with many other illnesses, the development of addiction is influenced by environmental conditions and behavior, but more heavily by the biological makeup of the individual. As with chronic pain, gender, age, ethnicity, social environment including cultural background, and conditions at work, home, and school can have an impact on addiction. Scientists estimate that genetic factors contribute between 40 and 60 percent of a person's vulnerability to addiction, while the effects of environment on gene expression and function are also significant. Furthermore, according to NIDA, "Adolescents and individuals with mental disorders are at greater risk of drug abuse and addiction than the general population."

One major biological/environmental factor that contributes to the development of the disease of addiction is having a family history of drug or alcohol abuse. This genetically predisposes a person to drug abuse. Another part of the puzzle as to what causes addiction is that starting to abuse a drug may lead to affiliation with more drug-abusing peers, which, in turn, exposes the individual to other drugs. Also, in a "permissive" household where it's okay to experiment with alcohol and other drugs, there is a higher incidence of drug use at an earlier age (cigarettes, alcohol, marijuana, and so on).

The more risk factors a person has, the more likely it is that the person will have abuse and addiction issues as time goes on. Some risk factors include early aggressive behavior, poor social skills, lack of parental supervision, substance abuse history, and poverty.

The risk of addiction can also depend on how you react to drugs. Basically, research has shown that those who have a negative reaction to drugs, such as nausea, dizziness, flushing, or confusion, are at a lower risk for addiction. Those who have a more positive reaction to the effects of drugs, like euphoria, anxiety reduction, or increased energy, are at a higher risk for developing addiction.

Drug abuse is, without question, one of the greatest health issues facing society today. Addiction reaches into every level of American life. Directly or indirectly, every family, every business, and every community is affected by drug addiction. Addiction is taking an unbelievable toll on our society.

Addiction to prescription drugs is a growing problem across the country. According to federal statistics, emergency-room visits caused by painkiller abuse have climbed more than 110 percent in the last seven years. Becoming addicted to painkillers is the manifestation of a disease. It is a disease of denial, and for some people who have a prescription drug problem, they don't realize or just don't want to admit it.

Addiction to alcohol, tobacco, and other drugs, and the health consequences of their use, is a widespread public health problem:

- One in four US hospital admissions is related to alcohol, tobacco, or other drug use.

- Of the more than two million deaths in the United States each year, approximately one in four is attributable to the use of alcohol, tobacco, or other drugs.

- Seventy-nine thousand deaths a year are due to binge drinking.

- One in four US children under the age of eighteen is exposed to an active case of alcohol abuse or dependence in the family. Countless numbers of children are adversely affected by parents and caregivers who are impaired by use of alcohol, tobacco, or other drugs.

- Treatment of patients with alcohol problems accounts for more than 15 percent of the national health care budget.

- Twenty-five percent of Medicare and 20 percent of Medicaid program expenditures are for treatment of the medical, surgical, and psychiatric complications of alcohol, tobacco, and other substance use and addiction.

Addicts often have other health problems, including mental disorders and diseases of the lungs, liver, kidneys, and brain as well as the cardiovascular system. Illegal drugs that are injected, such as heroin, cocaine, methamphetamine, and other drugs account for more than 30 percent of new AIDS cases. Injection drug use is also a major factor in the spread of hepatitis B and C, serious and potentially fatal liver diseases and a rapidly growing public health problem, according to NIDA. All drugs that are abused, legal as well as illegal, cause some form of intoxication, which interferes with judgment and increases the likelihood of risky sexual behaviors. This contributes to the spread of HIV, hepatitis B and C, and other sexually transmitted diseases. Furthermore, accidents and injuries increase dramatically for those who drive under the influence of mood-altering substances other than alcohol (drugged driving) because of decreased coordination and judgment and slowed reflexes.

Prescription drugs are increasingly being abused. This not only can lead to addiction, but can be fatal. NIDA, the Substance Abuse and Mental Health Services Administration (SAMHSA), and the Office of National Drug Control Policy (ONDCP) say that among the most disturbing aspects of this trend is its prevalence among teens and young adults. According to SAMHSA's *2009 National Survey on Drug Use and Health*, "3.1 percent of youths aged twelve to seventeen engaged in nonmedical use of prescription-type psychotherapeutics." Nonmedical use of prescription drugs occurred in 11.3 million Americans and was highest in eighteen-to-twenty-five-year-olds. It is a common misconception that prescription drugs are totally safe because they have been prescribed by a physician. In fact, 50 percent of these medicines are acquired by young people from the medicine cabinets of parents and friends. Furthermore, deaths from prescription opioid overdoses were second only to motor vehicle crash deaths among leading causes of unintentional injury death in 2007 in the United States. SAMHSA reported in a 2010 survey that the abuse of opioid painkillers had risen more than 400 percent over the last decade. This has resulted in a ramping up of efforts on a national level to modify that trend.

Treatment of Drug Addiction

Drug abuse and addiction are not death sentences, though if left untreated they can be fatal. There are treatment programs designed to help the addict become free of drugs and return to a healthy, more productive life. The sooner someone seeks help, the better his or her chances of recovery. Denying there is a problem is a classic symptom of addiction, so the first step involves admitting that drugs are having a negative impact on a person's life and that something must be done.

Many different treatments for addiction are available today. They include behavioral therapy, psychotherapy, counseling, medications, cognitive therapy, mutual help organizations, or combinations of all of these. They can occur in many different settings for varying lengths of time. Because addiction is a lifelong disease characterized by changes in the brain, successful treatment modalities in most cases also require a lifetime commitment. NIDA has formulated thirteen principles for effective addiction treatment. They are:

1 No single treatment is appropriate for all individuals.

2 Treatment needs to be readily available.

3 Treatment should attend to multiple needs of the individual, not just his or her drug use.

4 An individual's treatment plan must be assessed continually and modified as necessary to ensure the plan meets the person's changing needs.

5   Remaining in treatment for an adequate period is critical for treatment effectiveness.

6   Counseling and other behavioral therapies are critical components of effective treatment plans.

7   Medications are an important element of treatment for some, especially when combined with counseling and other behavioral therapies.

8   Addicted or other drug-abusing individuals with coexisting mental disorders should have both disorders treated in an integrated way.

9   Medical detoxification is only the first stage in addiction treatment and by itself does little to change long-term drug use.

10 Treatment does not need to be voluntary to be effective.

11 Possible drug use during treatment must be continually monitored.

12 Treatment programs should provide assessment for HIV/AIDS, hepatitis B and C, tuberculosis, and other infectious diseases, as well as counseling to help people modify or change behaviors that put themselves or others at risk of infection.

13 Recovery from drug addiction can be a long-term process and frequently requires multiple episodes of treatment.

The most effective treatments for addiction generally include a combination of different modalities because it is such a complex disease. The treatment modalities I include here are by no means the best or only methods for treating this debilitating problem.

Overview of Addiction Treatment

The treatment field has evolved since the 1950s, starting with the twenty-eight-day "Minnesota Model" and developing in many directions. Treatment for addiction can be provided in peer support settings, counselors' offices, outpatient programs, halfway houses, therapeutic communities, or inpatient programs. Most treatment programs provide a multidisciplinary approach that includes physicians, psychologists, social workers, counselors, nurses, family therapists, and support staff. They may incorporate any of the following treatment methodologies or combinations of therapies.

Since it is extremely difficult to remain abstinent from drugs, particularly opioids, and the relapse rate is high, many treatment professionals have turned to **medication-assisted treatment** (formerly called **maintenance**) that provides long-lasting opioids such as methadone or buprenorphine (Suboxone and Subutex). Today there are currently over 1,000 clinics authorized by the DEA to dispense methadone, a long-acting opioid that seems to cause less intoxication than other opioids. There are also over 1,800 treatment centers and over 12,000 physicians who are certified to prescribe buprenorphine. Buprenorphine causes fewer side effects than methadone and other opioids. With buprenorphine, there is less respiratory depression and cognitive impairment, and less euphoria, which is associated with craving and abuse.

There is abuse potential with methadone and buprenorphine, and that seems to limit their effectiveness for addiction treatment; however, many addicts have found their lives become more stable and their use of addicting drugs decreases. Others continue to abuse alcohol, stimulants, and even other opioids while they are using methadone or buprenorphine or between doses of these medications, which are being prescribed to help them stabilize their lives. Also, these medications don't help the addict with his or her life problems involving feelings, thoughts, relationships, and overall function.

If you are considering this form of treatment, I urge you to research it thoroughly before starting maintenance treatment. Both methadone and buprenorphine bind very tightly to the opioid receptor, resulting in extremely difficult withdrawal symptoms should you decide to discontinue them. Both medications are dangerous, especially if taken with sedatives such as alprazolam (Xanax) or diazepam (Valium) or others.

In the rest of this chapter, I will discuss models of treatment based on discontinuing the drugs and learning how to live without them. Effective treatments address cravings and relapse prevention, as well as learning how to cope with emotions and life situations that the drugs were used to treat.

The **Matrix Model** of treatment was initially designed to help stimulant abusers abstain from their drug of choice. It has since been expanded to include opioid and alcohol abuse. Patients are taught about addiction and relapse, receive direction and support from a trained therapist, become familiar with self-help programs, and are monitored for drug use. Most programs also include education for the addict's family.

In the Matrix Model the therapist acts as teacher and coach. The interaction between the therapist and the individual seeking treatment is realistic and direct, but not confrontational or parental. Therapists are trained to conduct treatment sessions in a way that promotes self-esteem, dignity, and self-worth. A positive relationship between patient and therapist is critical.

Motivational enhancement therapy is a client-centered approach to help those with addiction resolve ambivalence about engaging in treatment and stopping drug use. It is designed to use strategies evoking rapid internal changes, rather than guiding one through the recovery process. It consists of an initial assessment, followed by two to four individual treatment sessions with a therapist. Motivational interviewing principles are used to strengthen impetus and build a plan for change.

Supportive-expressive psychotherapy is a time-limited, focused psychotherapy with two main components including:

- Supportive techniques to help patients feel comfortable in discussing their personal experiences.

- Expressive techniques to help patients identify and work through interpersonal relationship issues.

Special attention is paid to the role of drugs in relation to feelings and behaviors and how problems may be solved without using drugs.

Individualized drug counseling focuses directly on reducing or stopping the patient's drug use. It addresses other issues that may be a problem such as employment issues, illegal activities, and family/social relations, as well as helping the patient initiate a recovery program. It helps the patient develop coping strategies and tools for abstaining from drug use, and then maintaining abstinence. The addiction counselor encourages twelve-step program participation and makes referrals for needed supplemental medical, psychiatric, employment, and other services.

Self-management and recovery training (SMART) is a secular and science-based recovery method using nonconfrontational motivational, behavioral, and cognitive forms of therapy. The program uses techniques found in motivational enhancement therapy and cognitive behavioral therapy. In SMART, addiction or substance dependency is viewed as a dysfunctional habit rather than a disease. SMART proponents allow that certain individuals may have a predisposition toward addictive behavior. It is based on four points in recovery, including:

- Building motivation.

- Coping with urges.

- Problem solving.

- Lifestyle balance.

Just as in twelve-step groups, local SMART chapters conduct meetings that are run by volunteers called "facilitators" with the assistance of volunteer recovery professionals called "volunteer advisors." It is generally listed as an alternative to twelve-step groups.

The SMART program:

- Teaches self-empowerment and self-reliance.

- Works on the obsessive and compulsive components of addiction as complex maladaptive behaviors with possible psychological factors.

- Teaches the use of tools and techniques needed for self-directed change.

- Encourages individuals to recover and live satisfying lives.

- Advocates the appropriate use of prescribed medications and psychological treatments.

- Evolves as scientific knowledge evolves.

Rational recovery (RR) is a self-help therapy started in 1988. It is based on the assumption that psychological difficulties, including addiction, are caused by irrational beliefs that can be understood and overcome through rational self-examination. RR members believe that planned abstinence is both desirable and possible. In RR, a coordinator conducts weekly or biweekly meetings with five to ten members. The coordinator maintains contact with a mental health professional "advisor" who is familiar with the RR program. The program emphasizes cognitive devices for abstinence.

Members use a "sobriety spreadsheet" on which they detail the irrational beliefs that activate their desire to use alcohol or other drugs. Members make a commitment to a planned, permanent abstinence from the undesirable substance or behavior, and then equip themselves with the necessary mental tools to stick to that commitment. The program is based on members recognizing and defeating the "addictive voice" and disassociating from addictive impulses.

Rational recovery:

- Regards alcoholism or addiction as a voluntary behavior as opposed to a disease.

- Discourages the adoption of the forever-recovering persona.

- Emphasizes self-efficacy.

- Has no distinct steps or any spiritual consideration.

Getting assistance that helps in long-lasting addiction recovery treatment is just as necessary as the early phases of addiction treatment. Recovery generally calls for a dedication to some type of program that ensures support and growth. No program can guarantee continuing addiction recovery, but research supports the belief that without such a program, ongoing recovery is much less likely to occur and be sustained.

Twelve-Step Programs

Twelve-step programs are the most successful and widely available treatment method for individuals seeking long-term recovery. Twelve-step programs use a mutual-support approach to recovery from addictive, compulsive, or other behavioral problems, based on adherence to a set of guiding principles. Originally developed in 1935 by the fellowship of Alcoholics Anonymous (AA) to help people recover from alcoholism, the way of life outlined in AA's Twelve Steps has been adapted to fit any number of manifestations of addiction and/or maladaptive behaviors. Because it has been such a successful methodology, the twelve-step model has expanded to include groups such as Narcotics Anonymous (NA), Cocaine Anonymous (CA), Crystal Meth Anonymous (CMA), Gamblers Anonymous (GA), Sex Addicts Anonymous (SAA), Codependency Anonymous (CODA), Emotions Anonymous (EA), and Overeaters Anonymous (OA), to name a few. These programs have helped millions of people worldwide to recover from the disease of addiction.

> *Twelve-step programs are the most successful*
> *and widely available treatment method for*
> *individuals seeking long-term recovery.*

Working the twelve steps includes:

- Admitting you can't control your addiction or compulsive behavior.

- Recognizing that a higher power can give you strength.

- Examining past mistakes with the help of a sponsor (someone who has been in the program for a while, has knowledge of the Twelve Steps, and can help explain the recovery process). Disclosing those mistakes is a powerful tool to decrease the shame and guilt many people feel after entering into recovery.

- Making amends for the mistakes.

- Learning a new code of behavior and living by it.

- Helping others who suffer from the same addiction or compulsive behavior.

The twelve-step approach involves group support from people who share their experience, strength, and hope for a better life outside addiction. All the different groups, which are usually organized at the local level, encourage regular participation. These groups put a lot of emphasis on spirituality, calling on the guidance of a "higher power."

Professional counseling is not a part of twelve-step programs. Attendees get guidance from other group members working on their own recovery and from sponsors, who are experienced group members.

The goal of twelve-step programs is abstinence from all mood-altering drugs, including the drug alcohol. Twelve-step programs stress the disease model of addiction. These programs have been shown to be an invaluable asset for anyone struggling to stay in recovery, especially when combined with other forms of treatment and counseling.

There is much new information about behavioral addiction (like gambling, spending/shopping, eating, and sex addiction) that is beyond the scope of this book.

Pain and Addiction

Many of the decisions about treating chronic pain with opioids are balanced against the risks of addiction. Of course, addiction is an extremely important consideration, but it should not be the only one. Part of the problem with addiction and pain treatment is due to confusion about the differences among the terms "tolerance," "physical dependence," and "addiction."

Because tolerance and physical dependence are to be expected with long-term use of opioids, it is easy for some to confuse these phenomena with addiction. Addiction is a disease that may require extended and exhaustive treatment; tolerance and dependence often can be successfully managed by the prescribing physician.

Dr. Richard Hanson explains that there are four goals that factor into the decision to use pain medications. They are:

1 **Reduce pain intensity.** It is not always realistic to expect medications to totally eliminate pain. More realistically, medication should be able to reduce pain to a level that is better tolerated.

2 **Improve ability to function.** Relief from pain often helps with a person's level of function. However, pain medications also can interfere with someone's ability to function.

3 Minimize adverse side effects. The goal is to find medications that maximize benefits while keeping side effects to a minimum.

4 Prevent addiction. No one likes the idea of getting addicted, and many fail to understand the dangers narcotic painkillers can have.

Many experts in the field of pain management, including Russell K. Portenoy, MD and Steven Passik, Ph.D., have referred to certain indications that might signal a possible problem with medication, including:

- Taking more medications, more often than was prescribed by the physician.

- "Doctor shopping," or attempting to get prescriptions from multiple doctors. There also may be repeated episodes of "lost" prescriptions.

- Aggressively complaining about the need for higher doses or requesting specific drugs.

- Hoarding or saving drugs during periods of reduced symptoms.

- Taking pain medications to deal with other problems such as stress.

- Stealing or "borrowing" medications from another patient.

- Engaging in concurrent abuse of related illicit drugs.

- Family members or others expressing concern about the person's use of pain medications.

If these behaviors are present, whoever is prescribing the medication should question whether addiction might be developing and discuss these concerns frankly with the patient. If you are using medications and having these experiences, perhaps it's time to discuss your concerns with your prescribing doctor.

Some people with chronic pain are vulnerable to addiction before they develop their pain. Once they are exposed to habit-forming medications, it is as if a switch is flipped and they lose control of their drug use, with increasingly negative results. If you have questions about your drug use for pain, I will attempt to help you understand some of the complex issues involved here.

As discussed in Chapter Four, opioids are one of the simplest and most efficient methods modern physicians have to treat severe chronic pain. There are over 500,000 prescriptions written every day for painkilling drugs to alleviate everything from headaches to severe sprains, to broken bones, to cramps, to long-lasting and debilitating chronic pain. They are preferred because they are so effective in controlling pain, they are easy to administer, and, in some cases, there are relatively few side effects. Generally, a doctor will prescribe the lowest possible dose of medicine for a patient in pain and then, if necessary, increase the amount gradually, in stages, until the pain is relieved or the opioids' side effects can no longer be tolerated. It is estimated that in 2010 about ten million patients were using opioids on a regular basis for chronic pain. This is ten times more than in 2000.

Opioids are not a panacea and are not appropriate for everyone. The use of these painkillers can be very dangerous.

> *Opioids are not a panacea and are not appropriate for everyone. The use of these painkillers can be very dangerous.*

For some people who have chronic pain, once the correct dose has been reached it remains effective for long periods of time, sometimes as long as the person requires medication, which may be indefinitely. In a large number of cases, however, people in pain develop tolerance and find they are taking higher and higher doses because their body adapts to taking opioids repeatedly over time, and it takes more of the drug to get the same painkilling effect. In some pain patients, if a higher dose becomes necessary, it might be because the disorder is getting worse, not that tolerance is developing, though either is a possibility and should be assessed by the prescriber.

It is necessary to understand, too, that a person may have demonstrated none of the outward signs usually associated with addiction, yet still become addicted to pain medication. According to Gourlay and Heit, the powerful painkillers many chronic pain patients take in order to function every day can have profound effects on their brains. Caution is in order when taking these medications, since some people tend to have a genetic predisposition to rapid tolerance and find, almost from the beginning that they are forced to take increasing amounts of medication to get the desired painkilling effect. Many discover that although they start with small doses of opioids, they quickly graduate to increasingly larger amounts and stronger medications. Some who have clear-cut histories of prior addiction to mood-altering drugs such as cocaine, methamphetamine, alcohol, marijuana, and others are at higher risk of becoming addicted to opioids.

Chronic pain causes many of the emotions that are also associated with addiction, such as fear, anxiety, depression, and unhappiness. This finding complicates an already murky picture.

This chapter is not meant to scare you from taking opioids or to warn you that if you take opioids for chronic pain you are just one pill away from addiction. There is absolutely nothing to substantiate the supposition of some people that if you must take strong painkillers, you will certainly become addicted. I am only attempting to point out the fact that there is *potential* for addiction if you use opioids, and just because you have a prescription for these medications from a doctor doesn't mean you are safe from addiction. Gourlay, Heit, et al., remind us in "Universal Precautions in Pain Medicine: A Rational Approach to the Treatment of Chronic Pain" that a careful assessment of the potential risks for using pain medications should be considered by your doctor, since prescription drug addiction can be devastating.

There are many signs that you may be on the threshold of an addiction problem. Some of the more common indicators include:

1   Continued use of the medication despite harm to you, physically or psychologically.

2   Withdrawal from family, friends, or social activities. Addiction often causes you to lose interest in many familiar activities and friendships. Family relationships also suffer.

3   Ignoring responsibilities such as work or school.

4   Increasing the dose of the drug. If you are addicted to painkillers you will begin to increase the amount of the drug you take without approval from your doctor.

5   Extending use. Despite recovering from the condition that initially caused the need for a painkiller, you continue to request and take the medicine. You may make the excuse that you are still in pain or need painkillers for a longer period, but you are actually taking them for an effect not intended by the prescribing doctor, such as anxiety relief or an energy burst.

6   Becoming defensive. You try to hide addiction, and you develop a tendency to become defensive and attack anyone who questions your drug use.

7   Being overly sensitive. Normally stressful situations suddenly become too hard for you to handle.

8   Personality changes. If you are addicted to painkillers, you may find that your normal behavior, energy, and mood may change.

9   Doctor shopping. You visit numerous doctors or emergency rooms to get prescriptions.

10 Forgetfulness. You may have trouble remembering things, especially things that have just happened.

11 Ignoring appearance and changing habits. You may begin to ignore personal hygiene. You also may have extreme changes in eating, exercise, and sleeping habits.

As discussed in Chapter Four, it is not unusual for those of you who have been taking prescription drugs for extended periods to find that once you stop the drugs, your pain diminishes. This is because the long-term use of opioids has caused a decrease in the ability to withstand pain and an increase in sensitivity to pain (opioid-induced hyperalgesia). This can lead you to think the painkillers are helping when in fact they make your pain worse. You may be surprised once you get the drugs out of your body and let your systems return to normal. You may have less pain than when you were taking the opioids.

Phyllis was clearly addicted to opioid painkillers as well as sedatives. She received most of the drugs by prescription from a few doctors, but she also was so tolerant that she had to buy them from friends and dealers. Thankfully, the elderly couple down the street was more than happy to sell their monthly script of Percocet to Phyllis at a lower cost than some of the local drug dealers. They had long ago decided that the side effects far outweighed the amount of pain reduction offered them by the Percocet—and the extra money was helpful to pay for groceries and rent. It was a win-win situation—except for Phyllis's liver. This organ was overburdened by the excessive doses of acetaminophen (Tylenol) in the huge number of pills she was taking in addition to the alcohol she drank to wash them down.

Her addiction showed up in many ways. She would crush the slow-release oxycodone (Oxycontin) tablets that were prescribed for her fibromyalgia and snort them for a more rapid onset of the effects. She was so physically dependent on the opioids that she came apart when she was down to her last thirty pills—anticipating the approaching end of her supply, running out and chasing more pills. And until she found them, she had to endure the stomach cramps, agitation, and anxiety that accompanied her almost weekly withdrawal.

But, she told herself, "I have to take these pills because I am in such pain from my fibromyalgia. I can't get out of bed if I don't swallow a few of these." Phyllis didn't see that she spent more time in bed than out, just like her mother had done. She rationalized her taking of pills and rejected people's attempts to help her. She stopped answering her Aunt Ellie's calls and cut herself off from most people, except those who could help her get drugs. Her meager inheritance from her father was quickly dwindling, and she wasn't sure what she'd do when it was all gone.

Phyllis's drug use and addiction finally came to a crisis point. By this time she was injecting methamphetamine, Oxycontin, and heroin. She had become tolerant to her prescription opioids, taking forty Percocet per day. To sleep, she took something every night, either two or three Lunesta, Valium, or Xanax, again having built up tolerance. She had been in detox twice, but suffered miserably in the withdrawal process and both times bolted after a few days in treatment to go get drugs.

When she ended up in the emergency room after an overdose, her aunt and several supportive friends confronted Phyllis in the form of a "mini-intervention." They pointed out Phyllis's behavior and physical deterioration, and expressed their sadness, concern, and fear that she would not recover and one day they would lose her to the disease of addiction. After several tearful hours, Phyllis agreed, once again, to enter treatment with a renewed commitment to trying to change her life. She was frightened and a bit hopeless, especially since she asked, "What about my pain?"

Phyllis personifies a most extreme example of the problems that occur when pain and addiction coexist—how one problem feeds the other, each making the other worse. Phyllis eventually realized, with her family's help, that the only way out was to detoxify from the habit-forming medications, which her body had become dependent upon. She then got treatment for the addiction that had gripped her mind, body, and spirit. Phyllis needed to take an honest look at her pain and figure out what to do about the body aches that caused her so much suffering. Eventually, she would find that her pain decreased simply in the process of detoxing and treating her addiction. She was well on her way to a better life, though you couldn't have gotten her to see it or believe it at the time.

If you are in pain, the threat of addiction is no reason to be denied all forms of treatment. It is important to understand, however, that opioids are potentially dangerous, and their use should be closely monitored. It is essential for your doctor to know if you're at high risk for addiction, such as if you have a personal or family history of drug abuse or if you suffer from emotional or mental problems. Certainly, if your history includes abusing drugs in any of the classes (stimulants, alcohol, depressants, marijuana, or opioids), you might well be at higher risk for developing a drug problem. In these cases, it might be wise to stick with alternatives to opioids, and if opioids are prescribed, to take them judiciously, with especially close monitoring. Use as little as possible, for as short a period as possible, and have someone hold and dispense the drugs. If you end up getting out of control, using more than intended, and/or continuing to use despite negative consequences, then you may be a person who simply cannot rely on opioids for pain relief. Also, if you are taking opioids, I strongly suggest not taking habit-forming sedatives or antianxiety drugs since these medications complicate the course of chronic opioid therapy.

In the hospital, Sam's attending doctor called in an addiction consultant whose wisdom and compassion touched Sam. The counselor had experience of her own with both recovery from addiction and chronic pain and really understood Sam's dilemma. He didn't identify as an addict since he had only used his medications as prescribed. He didn't get drugs on the street or crush and snort his medications, as he heard someone describe at a twelve-step meeting. Angela, his counselor, pointed out that the label of addict was so stigmatizing that Sam rejected it out of hand. She also helped him to see that he kept using the drugs despite the fact that they had stopped helping him long ago. He needed more over time and was clearly physically dependent, which required him to go through medically managed withdrawal in a local detox unit. His life and well-being revolved around the drugs and the meager pain reduction they offered. And his life was much worse on the drugs than off them. She encouraged him to look at and focus on the similarities rather than the differences between him and others he encountered with an addiction to drugs that looked very different from his in many ways.

With a lot of effort, he was able to see that the feelings associated with his drug use and how the effects of the drugs he used abated his awful emotional stresses. He felt angry at himself for being deformed and inadequate, and for isolating himself from others.

As you will see in the next chapter, dependence on medications has a negative effect on emotions that makes matters worse. You will benefit from working with your emotions whether or not you are taking medications. I wholeheartedly believe that until you address the emotional aspects of your chronic pain, your life will remain unsatisfying.

CHAPTER 6

"I Just Don't Feel Good . . ."

Emotions and Suffering

"When touched with a feeling of pain, the ordinary uninstructed person sorrows, grieves, and laments,

beats his breast, becomes distraught.

So he feels two pains, physical and mental.

Just as if they were to shoot a man with an arrow and, right afterward, were to shoot him with another one,

so that he would feel the pains of two arrows."

The Buddha

Suffering is feeling distress. It is a person's response to injury or loss. Suffering is the individual's response to a painful stimulus. It is unique for each individual and it involves emotions.

We all suffer sometimes in our lives, whether the suffering is physical, mental, emotional, spiritual, or a combination of all of these, as is often the case. Aristotle and Plato insisted that suffering (*pathos*) is a necessary part of the human condition. As human beings we *want* things, and when we don't get these things we feel badly. The more we want, the more disappointed we are when life doesn't go as we want.

More than 2,500 years ago, the Buddha taught in his "Four Noble Truths" that suffering exists, and it arises from attachment to desires. Suffering ceases when attachment to desire ceases and one can learn to be free. In other words, the less attached you are to certain things happening, for instance, getting a raise, falling in love, or being out of pain, the less you suffer.

As previously discussed, pain has many biological and psychological aspects. When you do something like stub your toe, get a splinter, or bump your head, you feel pain; it hurts. The acute pain will end and life will return to normal. With chronic pain, the pain goes on and on even after the splinter is out, or your toe is healed, or the lump on your head is gone. You begin to experience the hurt differently. Suffering is a major part of your experience with chronic pain. Humans respond with negative emotions, and matters always get worse when this happens.

Suffering is what you are feeling when you're angry because it hurts; when you get depressed because the pain won't stop; when you feel sad because you can't go out and play ball with the kids; when you are fearful that you won't be able to work and support your family; or when you feel hopeless because there seems to be little you can do to get better. Suffering is that element of chronic pain that is generated through your emotions. It describes moods characterized by sadness, anxiety, fear, irritability, anger, frustration, rage, guilt, shame, and loneliness.

These emotions are your *responses* to pain. They are generated from your attitudes, perceptions, memories, learned coping styles, and character traits. Some of how you react may be programmed into your genes. I've found that the reaction of some people to pain and their level of suffering are related to their predispositions and styles of responding to difficulties.

I Feel . . .

Many of you who must live daily with chronic pain are susceptible to creating and experiencing some of the emotions listed below. Just as when you have a bad day at work you are likely to get angry and unintentionally take out your frustrations on someone else, when you are in chronic pain you may also express your pain as unintentional anger or frustration. You develop a pattern of suffering and emotional pain. It often seems your life is about suffering and will always be about suffering. It is never-ending, inevitable, and intractable. There is no relief. You despair.

The following lists are not all-inclusive. There are many more; however, common feelings include:

- Anger
- Anxiety/Worry
- Sadness
- Fear
- Guilt
- Impatience
- Self-consciousness
- Irritation
- Frustration
- Love
- Shame
- Loneliness

In an effort to escape from the suffering of chronic pain, people often use defense mechanisms, which are unconscious psychological processes that come into play outside of your awareness to help you cope with painful aspects of reality. This process can happen quickly—sometimes in a matter of days or weeks—or unfold gradually over several months or even years. Common defense mechanisms include:

- Denial
- Rationalization
- Minimization
- Projection
- Aggression
- Deception
- Sarcasm
- Defiance
- Justification
- Judging
- Repression
- Withdrawal
- Humor

One of the most important things you can do to help yourself with your chronic pain is to develop insight into what you are feeling. Defense mechanisms prevent you from seeing what is true about your situation. For example, before he stopped using opioids, Paul couldn't do anything about his problem until he was able to *see* certain things. He was in denial that he was overusing drugs, and was consumed by guilt about the accident. He justified his drug use and irritability by rationalizing: "I have to take these drugs because of the pain. If you had my pain, you'd be taking these drugs too, Lila!" He withdrew from all of his support systems and repressed any feelings of anger at himself and God, though just under the surface he was seething with rage. He minimized his use, shouting, "I'm only taking what the doctor prescribed!" and neglecting to acknowledge the illegal marijuana he was smoking, the alcohol he was consuming, and the tendency he had developed to run out of his prescription a week early every month due to exceeding the daily allotted dose, leading him to buy drugs from his elderly neighbor who had cancer and would sell her medications to pay for food and rent.

In other words, Paul's emotions were a mess. In order to shift out of his downward spiral, he needed to see his process more clearly, which was difficult for him to do while drugs were clouding his mind and his defense mechanisms were obscuring the pain of his reality.

Awareness Is the Key

Insight and knowledge about what you are thinking and feeling are essential to making changes. There are many techniques to practice in order to increase self-awareness. One psychological tool is the **Johari Window**, created by Joseph Luft and Harry Ingham in 1955. The idea is that there are four "rooms" or "quadrants" in your life. One room is the one that is known to you and others, which is "open" or the "arena." There is part of you that is known to others but not to yourself, called the "blind spot." You learn about your blind areas by hearing information or feedback from others who see what you do not. Another room is called the "façade," which represents the part of you that you know but others don't. You can shrink this area by telling people things they do not know and cannot see about you. Finally, the fourth room is unknown to you *and* to others. This is truly the unconscious part of you that can be revealed as you communicate with others and accept honest feedback. As you learn more, you become more self-aware and can use this knowledge to make necessary changes to improve your life.

Example of the Johari Window

	Known to Self	Unknown to Self
Known to Others	My Public Self	My Blind Spots
Unknown to Others	My Hidden Self	My Unconscious Self

There are many ways to help you cope with your emotions and see what is true, what is really going on. Counselors, psychologists, therapists, clergy, doctors, and even a trusted friend or family member can provide feedback to you about what they are seeing. Your work is to accept the feedback as information and not judgment. Often, the closer a person is to you, the harder it may be for him or her to give you feedback that is not laced with judgment or recrimination. When Lila shouted back at Paul, "You're nothing but a loser and an addict! You are not the man I married!" it became almost impossible for Paul to respond with anything but defensiveness.

> *Insight and knowledge about what you are thinking and feeling are essential to making changes.*

On the other hand, Paul's pain doctor sat with him and gently pointed out the patterns that were developing: "Paul, I'm concerned about you because you are running out of your prescriptions earlier each month, which indicates to me that you are becoming tolerant to your medications. Also, you tested positive for marijuana in your urine, so let's talk about the fact that you are supplementing legal pain medications with illegal ones. It seems like you have a better relationship with the pills than you do with me. Every time I see you, you look stoned and not shaved or showered. When I see this pattern, I don't think our treatment plan for your pain is effective. I'd like to talk about alternatives, including coming off your medications and seeing what happens. How do you feel about that?" Because Paul's doctor had a more objective overview of what was going on with Paul, he was able to discuss options in a nonjudgmental manner. Paul was able to listen because he didn't feel he was being judged. And though the fear of giving up the only relief he had in his difficult life was overwhelming, deep down he knew the doctor was right, and he started to think that he might want to try what the doctor suggested. This was the beginning of Paul's recovery.

The Link Between Your Emotions and Your Suffering

Just as chronic pain is unique, how you experience and react to chronic pain is based on who you are—how you were raised, your previous experiences with pain, and your thoughts and feelings about chronic pain. These emotional reactions can change week to week, day to day, and often moment to moment. For many of you, there really is no way to predict what you'll be feeling each day. There are emotional aspects of chronic pain that contribute to your experience. They include:

1   Your outlook on pain in general.

2   Your personal history.

3   How severely you feel pain—your pain thermostat, e.g., central pain.

4   How you believe it will affect your life.

5   The reactions of your family and friends to your pain.

It is important for you to understand that emotional pain is very much a part of chronic pain. The emotions you experience in your responses to pain *contribute* to suffering; they are part of the hurt you feel from chronic pain. There is extensive research proving that those who have sustained an acute injury and who also have suffered from some sort of trauma shortly before the acute problem are more likely to develop chronic pain than those who have not been emotionally or physically traumatized. And for those of you in chronic pain, you know you experience more physical pain when you are also in emotional pain.

Think about a day when you had an especially difficult time sleeping. You might have been awakened by your pain and were unable to get back to sleep. As you lay in bed, you became more and more frustrated. You desperately needed sleep, but the pain wouldn't stop. It nagged and pulled and pushed and throbbed. All you could think of was everything you had to do the next day. The stress began to build and build and you began to hurt more and more.

Then you got angry. Your heart began to pound, your muscles tightened, and you began to toss and turn more. Suddenly, you found your pain had increased and sleep now was totally out of the question. You were forced to get up and give up sleeping altogether. Whether you realized it at the time or not, you had succeeded in *making yourself feel worse;* you increased your own pain and caused yourself more suffering!

Now think about a night when, for whatever reason, you slept well, or at least better than you normally sleep. You got a good six hours of sleep. You were stiff and sore when you awoke because you slept for so long, but when you arose you were rested. You actually felt encouraged that you would be able to do all the things you had set out for yourself. It was a marvelous feeling. Your coffee tasted hot and good, and your morning shower was refreshing. Of course, you still had pain, but it didn't seem to be quite so important. You weren't suffering as much. This is an example of how your positive attitude had affected your pain positively, resulting in less pain. This means your good mood and optimistic feelings lessen your pain.

What these two examples illustrate is that your emotions have an impact on your pain. Negative emotion increases pain. Positive emotion decreases pain. More pain equals more suffering. Furthermore, when you *resist* the pain, the pain increases. When you *relax* into the pain and stop fighting it, you feel less suffering. Increased resistance increases pain. Decreased resistance decreases pain.

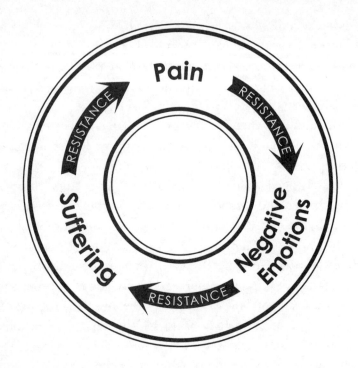

Feelings: Annoyance, Frustration, Anger, Resentment, and Rage

These emotions run on a spectrum from mild to intense. Usually all are attached to not getting what you want or fear of having something taken away. (See the section on fear on page 90.)

Anger is a normal emotion and part of the response system charged with protecting you from getting hurt. It is part of the alert system in the brain managed by the sympathetic nervous system. This function is one humans share with animals. The human version of anger is complex and is involved with your needs and expectations not being met in addition to getting your feelings hurt (disappointment).

When you are in pain it is common to direct anger at yourself, even at the specific site of the physical pain—"My darned back is hurting again." You send these angry thoughts and feelings through your nervous system to the site of the pain, and the pain gets worse. You may direct anger at yourself because you are unable to do the things you would like to do or, just as commonly, at others who are close to you, such as family members and friends, for "not understanding" or "not being supportive."

It is equally common for you to be angry with the medical system, specifically the doctors who were unable to help you or who prescribed the medications that you became dependent on, or the insurance company that won't let you get the next procedure or see the next doctor or pay you enough for your disability.

Sometimes you are angry at one thing but your anger is manifested elsewhere. For example, you think, "The truth is I'm mad because my back hurts," but you shout at your son and punch the wall. This is called displaced anger.

What to do about anger? First and foremost, you must know that you are angry; you must develop awareness about your anger and the fact that it exists. It is only by being aware that you have any chance of changing the damaging effects of persistent, cultivated anger, which can be called resentment. Unchecked, anger can progress to rage—commonly termed "seeing red" or "losing it"—a loss of self-control that often leads to violence against oneself or others.

Next, you need to ascertain what you are really angry about; the true reason you are angry. Once you're aware that you are angry and begin to figure out where the anger is actually coming from, you then can address the true cause of your anger. You can develop a set of skills and tools to address these feelings. Knowing the source of the anger is helpful, as is looking beneath the apparent reason of "He's just a jerk" to a deeper level of "My feelings were hurt."

With awareness comes the ability to apply techniques to slow down the progression of anger, such as the proverbial "counting to ten" or breathing and getting in touch with the rapid heartbeat, flushed feeling, and discomfort in your head. Writing about your feelings can be very helpful in unraveling the complex web of emotions you become trapped in. Also, talking to someone who is supportive and knowledgeable can be invaluable in helping you cope with anger. Turning to a higher power, as you understand the concept of a higher power, can assist you in unraveling the maelstrom of angry feelings. Forgiveness of others and yourself is an extremely helpful practice to relieve anger. Finally, talking with a professional, for example, a counselor, psychologist, or medical professional, can often help you sort things out as you address your anger.

Fear

Fear can be pervasive and all-encompassing, and very frequently is the feeling that underlies anger. It is commonly associated with avoiding what we are afraid of. Dr. Jodie Anne Trafton presents research that has proven that when someone is afraid, his or her pain scores increase. Conversely, teaching people to reduce their fear about a situation can decrease their pain.

For example, you may tell yourself, "If I sit too long at the movies, I'm afraid that my neck is going to kill me. I know because it always does." Notice the power of such a statement. It becomes a prediction and it happens. On the other hand, you can tell yourself, "This movie is going to be so good, my neck doesn't have to be as sore. I'll get up when I have to and stretch. The discomfort will be worth it for the laughs." These thoughts can reduce the amount of pain you experience. Rehearsing the activity with a positive attitude reduces the fear. "I'll get an aisle seat. When I get uncomfortable, I'll simply get up and walk around. Missing a few minutes of the movie is preferable to not going at all." Even more surprising is that brain activity in the area where pain is experienced, the cingulate gyrus in this case, decreases when fear diminishes.

Fear Avoidance

It is common with an injury that results in chronic pain to develop a number of fears. Take a minute to think about what you are afraid of. Are you afraid that:

- You'll die?

- You'll be unhappy and unable to escape?

- You won't be able to handle it?

- You'll hurt yourself?

- You don't deserve this, and it won't work?

- If you feel pain, it means you're harming your body and making matters worse (hurt vs. harm)?

- Moving, which causes you to hurt, means something is wrong inside, and you must protect yourself by moving less?

- If you exercise, the pain will increase to uncontrollable levels?

- You will never be able to function the way you used to (walk, lift your baby, ski, or sit in a movie), so you'd rather not try and be disappointed?

These are irrational fears. When you believe these fears, you avoid doing things that, in the long run, are good for you, like moving and exercising and not taking a pill. The net effects are that you become deconditioned from not moving and it becomes harder to move because you're not used to it. You rest and avoid normal activities until "normal" becomes a "frozen" way of living—physically and emotionally.

Paul found that whether he moved or not, his pain was there. Resting only made him weaker and more depressed. The less he moved, the more afraid he was of moving, and in fact, the less he could move, and the more he hurt. As he began to exercise with a trainer, Paul noticed, to his surprise, that his pain didn't get any worse. His worst fears were proven untrue. Even more surprising and exciting was that after he was working out regularly, his pain diminished substantially.

Sam found that when he was angry, his pain would flare. He didn't realize it at first, but after talking with a counselor he noticed the effect of this emotion on his perception of pain. And Sam was angry a lot. He experienced anger toward his parents, his boss, his coworkers, the doctors who advised him badly—first by "botching" his surgery and then by prescribing medications without warning him of how they would affect him. He was angry at his girlfriend for dumping him, angry at God for cursing him with his rotten body, and angry at himself for not having the courage to end it all.

At the same time, his fear was pervasive. He feared that he would never find love again, that he would end up being crippled in a wheelchair, that the medications would permanently ruin his ability to concentrate, and that he would lose the thing about himself that he valued the most: his keen mind. He also feared getting injured, and stayed away from any activity that might cause him to be hurt. He feared exercising because it made him hurt more, and his inactivity caused him to be less able to move. His world shrunk; he felt worse about himself, and the net result was that he felt more pain.

Paul had so much guilt about the accident that he could barely stand to be awake. The face of the girl who died in the accident came to him in his dreams and whenever the drugs and alcohol wore off. In those moments, he thought he would surely die of shame and remorse for causing so much harm to another human and her family. He also had an incredible amount of guilt about Lila and his son, feeling he had let them down as a husband, father, and breadwinner. He was impotent from all the drugs he used and felt guilty about that as well.

Both Paul and Sam were depressed and consumed with a sense of hopelessness and helplessness. They had a sense that things would never get better; in fact, they both were convinced things would likely get worse. Paul was panicked after his recent visit to the doctor at the thought of giving up all of his mediations; after all, "How can I possibly get through the day without my drugs?" On those occasions when Paul and Sam were able to think more positively about their respective situations, each experienced a small bit of relief from their chronic pain.

In fact, one study shows that just the expectation that something can ease your pain will actually do it. In this study, a salve was applied to the bodies of people in pain. They were told that the salve was a pain reliever and would help them. EEGs taken during the experiment revealed that when the people in the study thought they were getting an analgesic,

Cycle of Uncontrolled Pain and Fear

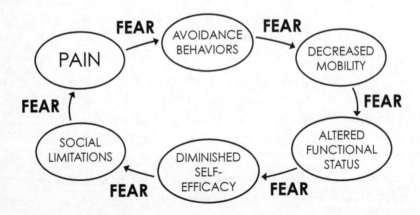

their brain's pain centers showed reduced activity and they reported less pain. In another study, subjects were told that pressing a lever quickly enough would reduce the pain level from an electric shock. Most people in the study said the shock was not as painful when they thought they were fast enough, even though the lever was connected to nothing. So belief about what will happen can make it happen.

The Placebo Effect

It is well-known that beliefs arise in your brain and in your mind. Those beliefs and the emotions associated with them have lasting and profound effects on your body. The power of the mind to help you deal with chronic pain has been documented many times over. One of the most dramatic confirmations of this is illustrated by the placebo effect. The placebo effect occurs when you improve or get better simply by believing that a treatment or medication is going to help you improve or get better. Patients who are given inactive substances and told these substances will take away their pain respond to the placebo at least 25 percent of the time.

Placebos work even though they shouldn't. The only explanation is that your belief causes the effect in your body through neurotransmitter activation caused by your beliefs. You have amazing power to heal yourself if you only believe you can.

One study of the placebo effect involved heart patients who received surgery to eliminate angina (chest pain). During the operation, the internal mammary artery was to be tied off to theoretically help the heart grow new blood vessels and increase the blood flow to the heart muscle, which would, in turn, decrease the patient's chest pain. The results of this placebo-controlled trial were published in *The New England Journal of Medicine*. Of seventeen patients, eight had the actual operation. The other nine were anesthetized and received simple incisions, but nothing else. The fake or placebo operations worked as well as the real operations. The patients' belief that the surgical procedure was done and would help decrease chest pain actually caused clinical improvement (reduction of chest pain). This is a perfect example of the power of one's beliefs causing improvement in a physical condition. These patients thought they were going to get better after surgery, and they did. In other words, your mind controls your body.

Another study showed that in patients who had arthritis of the knee, surgically scraping out the knee joint had results comparable to those of people whose knee joint was simply opened and closed without the scraping procedure. Unfortunately, there has been little research involving the placebo effect when discussing conventional back pain treatments, including surgery.

Several studies have reported that a person's beliefs about how well treatment for chronic pain would work before it was started influenced how well the treatment worked. This is called **treatment expectancy**—the stronger the expectancy, the better the outcome. Conversely, expecting to be anxious about a particular act results in anxiety. When Paul finally came to believe that "this will work," he found that the treatment interventions worked. Until he believed in the process, he suffered more and more, needlessly. Believing something will work makes it work.

Dr. Stephen Colameco says too much emphasis is placed on the belief that chronic pain is purely a physical response to a stimulus and not enough attention is paid to social and psychological influences. Chronic pain is very often the result of mental, not physical, processes.

Colameco says he believes the medical model of chronic pain treatment "may reinforce patients' beliefs that 'the' cause of pain can be isolated to an anatomic abnormality or injury, potentially contributing to the 'sick role' and consequently delaying effective behavioral treatments."

It has also been shown that when the minds of people in pain were distracted by something that required intense concentration, their brains' pain centers demonstrated decreased activity. This means that when you are distracted from the pain, it hurts less. You may have experienced this yourself. You get involved in an interesting conversation or are watching a riveting ball game on television and you get distracted and forget your pain, or in fact, you actually *don't feel the pain*. My pain routinely diminishes when I lecture unless I call attention to it.

All too often, when you experience chronic pain, your sensory system goes on automatic pilot. You become so consumed with feeling the pain that you lose the ability to stand back and look at the experience from a different perspective. The pain may be so intense and overwhelming that it is impossible to think of anything else. It is at these moments that you are more likely to feel anxious, stressed, angry, depressed, unhappy, frustrated, or helpless. Your emotions begin to run full throttle, contributing to the worsening of your pain because of your suffering.

Pain is definitely influenced by your beliefs about it. In my clinical practice, I have observed again and again that when people develop trust that a process will help—especially if they are open to the process helping and are motivated to improve—they invariably note an improvement, that is, a decrease in their pain and improvement in their mood. The power of your beliefs can transcend physical conditions and often results in marked improvement in your level of pain, and certainly in a decrease in the amount you suffer.

Secondary Gain

There are certain forces that will hold you back in the process of letting go of your pain. First ask yourself: "What/who would I be without my pain?" It might be a challenge to answer that question since your pain has been with you for so long. Maybe you've even forgotten who you are. For some of you, pain has become your identity. The pain drives you, motivates you, restricts you, hurts you (physically, emotionally, mentally, and spiritually), aggravates you, frustrates you, preoccupies you, angers you—in other words, pain has become your life. Your pain holds you hostage. You become caught in a cycle of chaos, longing for freedom from the hurt and not knowing how to take the first step toward breaking free. The longer you go around and around, the bigger the circle becomes, until the pain affects everything and everyone in your life. You find yourself standing alone—lost and afraid that you'll never be the same again.

Oddly enough, an interesting thing happens at this point. Because pain is now "who you are," you may want to guard that identity. You may find there are certain benefits to being in pain. Let's try an experiment. Take a deep breath and, without thinking, list all of the advantages of having chronic pain. Remember to suspend your judgments. Some people come up with a number of surprising items on their lists. If totally honest and uncensored, they list things like:

- It gets me attention from others.

- It is a steady and consistent part of my life. I can count on it.

- It is familiar.

- It gets me out of doing things I'd rather not do.

- It keeps me from feeling other things or feelings.

- It gives me an excuse to be angry, withdrawn, isolated.

- It gives me an excuse to take drugs.

About now, some of you may be twisting this page of the book and thinking, "Are you crazy? There's nothing good about the *%#!*$% pain!"

The human organism responds to rewards, and in fact, there are benefits you receive from your pain and the behaviors associated with it, though more often than not these behaviors are not willful, intentional, or conscious. The items listed above are known as **secondary gain**. Even though this phenomenon may be an entirely unconscious action on your part, you gain something by staying stuck in this cycle of helplessness and dysfunction. Knowledge about how secondary gain works in your life can lay the foundation for an insightful release from these potentially destructive behaviors. If you are truthful with yourself, you will learn interesting information that will help you get better.

As you read this, please try not to be judgmental about what you learn. Try to be interested in the information, curious as to how these benefits have developed and how they affect you.

Avoiding the Feelings

Many of you with chronic pain have inadvertently developed a pattern of avoiding emotions. You do your best to ignore and deny these feelings because they are so unpleasant. They never go completely away, however. These feelings hover just out of sight, casting a dark shadow of misery. They still cause problems. By ignoring them, you are allowing these negative feelings free range over your mood and experience, and you become a victim of the very thing you are fighting not to have. You expend a lot of effort attempting to avoid the things you label unpleasant, undesirable, or unwanted. Contrary to intentions and expectations, consciously or unconsciously, the harder you resist, the more you suffer.

Contrary to intentions and expectations,
consciously or unconsciously,
the harder you resist, the more you suffer.

Growing Awareness Is Powerful

Emotions affect one's experience of pain from moment to moment. Phyllis went to visit her pain management doctor with a changed look on her face. As the meeting began, she reported that the previous day, by utilizing breathing techniques and a massage, her pain was down to five out of ten. She looked rather pleased as she described this experience. Then she said that at the moment, her pain was her usual eight out of ten, but acknowledged—somewhat reluctantly—that she had had a dispute with the cable company earlier that morning. She was still irked that she couldn't get a charge reversed.

"But let's get back to yesterday," her doctor said. "You said your pain was a five out of ten most of the day, right?" Phyllis scrunched up her face and reported, "It was *only* yesterday," implying the relief had come and gone, thereby minimizing its significance.

The doctor gently nudged her toward the truth. "Your pain was a five out of ten for most of the day, and you took no medications. We call that a breakthrough, Phyllis!"

She would have missed it—naturally induced relief as effective as or actually more effective than her medications. Previously she only would get to a six out of ten after taking all of her medication, and on the doses she took, she would sleep most of the day. Her doctor pointed out the converse: Her pain had risen dramatically in direct relation to the dispute with the cable company. In fact, as she and her doctor spoke, Phyllis had a distinct lessening of her pain as she saw the nature of the anger and let it go. After all, the overcharge was just $2.99. Just like that, her suffering diminished. The fact that this happened filled Phyllis with a tremendous feeling of well-being. She experienced a sense of optimism that she was able to do this and that this actually could work.

"Wow, I've wasted so much time under the influence of medications and have had so much unnecessary suffering because of my anger," Phyllis said. In that moment, her pain rose a bit as she found herself fretting and nibbling on her lower lip. As she realized what she was doing, she took a few deep, cleansing breaths and her pain started to ease again. Armed with a new sense of power and self-efficacy, Phyllis thanked her doctor and left. She felt exhilarated.

Becoming aware of what you are feeling and trying honestly and calmly to assess what is happening can help you cope with your pain. Recognizing that you are angry, depressed, or stressed out because of your pain may mean you can exert some control over the level of pain affecting you. This is where mindfulness practice can be extremely informative and helpful. You will notice that just paying attention to what you are feeling changes the feeling. Being willing to acknowledge and accept your emotions and feel them as they arise may help remove their negative power.

I'm not trying to say that if you admit that you're angry because of chronic pain, the soreness or aching are going to disappear. I am saying that if you must live with chronic pain, you can benefit from being attentive to your emotional well-being, and *your experience of pain will change*. If you get good at this—by practicing regularly—you will have an effective tool at your disposal to decrease your suffering.

For many in chronic pain, life is a daily grind of relentless agony. The sustained pain seems endless, slowly wearing you down until there seems to be nothing left but the pain. Your daily pain level may hit a six or seven or eight on a scale where ten is the worst pain you've ever experienced.

Now imagine you can change that six or seven or eight to a five or six or seven, just by changing your emotional outlook. Wouldn't it be worth it if you could reduce your pain level by even 10 percent just by recognizing that you are angry because you hurt or that anxiety is creeping up on you because of the pain? Wouldn't it be great if you made your pain less by even one notch just by believing today is going to be better than yesterday?

It's possible and it's real, and I have seen it happen again and again. By simply looking at his anger, Paul could diminish it, and by diminishing his anger he could lessen his pain.

Sam learned that when he faced his fear, noticing what he was afraid of and what was *really* going on, his pain diminished. Phyllis began to loosen her hold on controlling everything in her life to make up for her not being in control of so much in her life for so long, and the pain's hold on her decreased.

There are many ways to take an active part in reducing your pain. In the chapter on treatment modalities you find many of them, including yoga, meditation, Pilates, aromatherapy, and many more. Imagine the results you might get by really applying some of the suggested methods in this book.

One challenge for you is that you need sustained effort to effect sustained change. In other words, take a pill, and once it takes hold the effect will last a few hours or more. The pill is reliable, if imperfect, in its efforts. It does relieve the pain. On the other hand, the benefits of the techniques discussed in this chapter may last only as long as you can hold your attention on them, but then you can restart the effort—again and again in each moment. If you practice and get better at holding the attention for longer periods, you get more sustained relief.

What have you got to lose but your pain?

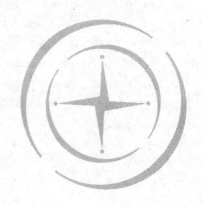

CHAPTER 7

Working with Thoughts and Emotions

"Pain is not a punishment. Pleasure is not a reward."

Pema Chödrön

Emotions and thoughts are at the root of chronic pain for many people. To cope effectively with chronic pain, it is important to pay attention to both thoughts and emotions and learn to notice and eventually modify them. In essence, the way you think and feel affects your pain. Learning to work with thoughts and emotions gives you a handle on how to control your pain.

Many people shun the idea of working with thoughts and emotions— suggesting that this means the pain "is all in my head." My response to those folks is: "Where else do you think it is?" Perhaps not all, but the vast majority of the pain experience, and consequently your ability to affect and ultimately reduce pain, lies with your thoughts and emotions. If the only work you are doing is to attend to the *sensation* of the pain and you don't address the rest of the experience—the suffering—you are missing the most important work you can do with the ways you think and feel about the pain. And the work allows you to make a significant impact on your experience of pain. It gives you more control of your experience of pain.

From Comfortable with Uncertainty *by Pema Chödrön. © 2002 by Pema Chödrön and Emily Hilburn Sell. Reprinted by arrangement with Shambhala Publications, Inc., Boston, MA. www.shambhala.com.*

There is a tremendous variability in the ways in which people cope with pain and its consequences. Your beliefs and attitudes are the most important components in your ability to change your perceptions of your pain and thus diminish your suffering.

> *Your beliefs and attitudes are the most important*
> *components in your ability to change your perceptions*
> *of your pain and thus diminish your suffering.*

In the last chapter, I reviewed those emotions that typically affect chronic pain. Now, what are you going to do about them? There are many therapeutic techniques that have been proven to help individuals with chronic pain. This chapter will review three commonly used interventions: cognitive behavioral therapy (CBT), acceptance and commitment therapy (ACT), and mindfulness meditative practices. All three methods are geared to enhancing the function of the parasympathetic nervous system and diminishing the high levels of sympathetic nervous system activation. As you will see, there are many similarities among these therapies, and each builds on the others.

Cognitive Behavioral Therapy (CBT)

Cognitive behavioral therapy is a form of psychotherapy based on the idea that thoughts and not external things cause feelings and behaviors. CBT therapists believe that by changing the way you think, you can change how you feel and act. In CBT, therapists help you first identify negative and distorted thought patterns, and then replace them with positive thoughts. Unlike many psychotherapy methods that focus on past conflicts, CBT concentrates on observing and then changing current and future behaviors. CBT techniques vary according to the client or issue(s) the client is having. In general, however, CBT is based on methods developed in behavior and cognitive therapies.

Behavioral therapy stresses positive reinforcement, in which positive behavior is rewarded, and desensitization, in which you confront the things that cause fear, discomfort, and anxiety and then overcome these negative emotions. In cognitive therapy, you identify distorted thought patterns, which are called "maladaptive schema," and replace them with more constructive ones. This is called "cognitive restructuring."

Your thought patterns, reactions, and beliefs about pain greatly influence your perception of pain. You can change painful feelings by using mental tools to alter your thoughts about your pain. CBT teaches that you cannot change or control other people or situations, but you can control the way you react to a situation.

CBT therapists understand that pain is much more than just the body's biological response to a stimulus. The perception of pain includes such things as previous painful episodes, stress, fears, anxiety, sadness, depression, and other moods. CBT therapists design treatments to teach you that your perception of pain is related to your thoughts, and thoughts can be controlled and modified. You can learn how to think differently and then act on that learning.

There is evidence that CBT works better than taking medication long-term in the treatment of chronic pain. CBT has been successfully used for people with back and neck pain, headaches, arthritis, fibromyalgia, insomnia, chronic fatigue syndrome, lupus, abdominal and chest pain, sickle cell anemia, and cancer, among other disorders. CBT can be divided into two parts, "functional analysis" and "skills training." In the first part, the therapist and you identify the stressful problem. Then a determination is made about which thoughts might lead to or worsen the problem. If the thoughts and reactions are deemed inappropriate or unhelpful, the therapist will help you unlearn the unwanted reactions and learn appropriate helpful reactions.

Some common patterns of negative thinking that CBT therapists seek to change include:

- Generalizing: looking at an event as the start of a never-ending cycle.

- Personalizing: accepting blame automatically when something bad occurs and feeling like it's "all about me."

- Polarizing: insisting on viewing or seeing situations as all black or all white, with no shades of gray.

- Catastrophizing: anticipating the worst and exaggerating perceived failures and symptoms, especially in regard to chronic pain.

- Filtering: exaggerating the negative aspects of a situation and minimizing the positive ones.

CBT seeks to help you get beyond these negative ways of thinking. CBT tries to help you change your views of the world from overwhelming thoughts. Many therapists emphasize maintaining a level of composure—remaining as calm and balanced as possible no matter what the degree of reaction.

- Cool thoughts are usually simple statements of fact. No particular emotion is suggested by these statements. "Most days I have chronic pain."

- Warm thoughts are linked to a mild degree of reaction and typically are associated with preferences. It's normal to be distressed when situations or events don't happen as you would like. "I wish I didn't have to hurt today."

- Hot thoughts are associated with intense emotions and significant distress such as panic, heavy depression, or intense anger, out of proportion to the situation. "If I have to continue living in chronic pain, I'd rather be dead." Often, it is not the situation that causes all the emotional distress; it is the person's thoughts about the situation.

In these examples, the CBT practitioner would try to teach the client to substitute warm thoughts for hot thoughts, as Paul had learned that slowing his breathing could diminish some of his hurt. His ultimate frustration and anger led him to the hot thought, "I'd be better off dead." This thought was tempered, once his breath slowed, by the truth, a cooler thought: "This pain will subside. It always does. I can make it better or worse. The choice is up to me." As Paul's muscles relaxed, his pain diminished in that moment and his thoughts shifted from hot to warm and finally to cool. "It's a beautiful day, and after my massage I'm going to go for ice cream with Lila and William."

According to Dr. Richard Hanson, the primary goals of CBT are to:

1   Identify unrealistic, distorted, self-defeating, and irrational thoughts and beliefs that create more distress and misery than necessary.

2   Challenge and dispute these irrational thoughts and beliefs.

3   Develop more healthy beliefs and attitudes.

4   Increase the confidence that you have the ability to successfully manage adverse situations and events. You can cope with difficult situations by applying learned problem-solving techniques.

CBT helps you to change your thought processes and focus on doing things for yourself in positive ways. Therapists operate on the assumption that emotional and behavioral reactions to pain are learned and therefore can be unlearned.

You may benefit in many ways from CBT therapy. Some of the more obvious benefits include:

- Improved pain management—truly less pain, and certainly less suffering.

- An increased belief in your own capability to successfully handle life's problems—a sense of self-efficacy: "I can do that!"

- Lowered stress level. Heightened ability to relax.

- A better quality of life.

- Better relationships with others.

Although CBT takes less time than other forms of psychotherapy, success is not something that happens overnight. Generally, the CBT therapist and the client meet for between five and twenty sessions, each one lasting between thirty and ninety minutes. During the first few sessions, the client and therapist join forces to identify the client's problem, discuss the goals the client wants to achieve out of the therapy, and discuss ways to reach those goals. It is a collaborative effort.

According to the National Association of Cognitive-Behavioral Therapists (NACBT), therapists do not tell clients what their goals should be or what they should tolerate. Rather, they interact with the client and show him or her how to think and behave in a way that will enable the client to reach his or her desired goals. Therapists don't tell their clients what to do so much as explore and discover what the clients want and then teach them how to get it.

Therapists often distinguish between healthy and unhealthy responses to situations. Responses typically are seen as unhealthy when they are extreme emotional reactions, totally out of proportion to reality. Additionally, for pain clients, when a reaction is self-defeating and causes more pain, it is also considered unhealthy. The varying degrees of these unhealthy reactions have been labeled as "cool," "warm," or "hot." For example, when you are in chronic pain and catastrophize, you see your life as nothing more than a painful condition that will only get worse. CBT helps with these "hot thoughts" by teaching you that although you may be in pain—this and every moment—it can be managed. It is not a hopeless condition and need not consume you or necessarily get worse. These "cool thoughts" diminish suffering.

After Sam stopped taking medications, he still had significant pain and many of the problems associated with that pain, including depression, anxiety, and anger about his condition and his lot in life. CBT taught him that changing his thoughts and identifying his negative feelings could help him cope with not just his emotional distortions, but the pain that had caused them.

Through CBT Sam learned to work on negative thoughts when his pain flared up. Typically, during times when the pain was especially bad, as it often got throughout his day, Sam would anxiously try to rush to get things done before he felt incapacitated. He eventually learned that the anxiety and rushing through life were making the pain worse. The stress and tension of living were increasing his suffering, which in turn created more anxiety, pain, and so on. Relaxing and slowing down helped Sam ease his tension, thereby easing his pain. Thinking differently about his pain also was helpful. After all, it slowed him down, and as he slowed down he began to appreciate the world around him ("cool thoughts")— the mountains in the background, a breeze across his face, the sound of his favorite symphony. As he slowed down and breathed, joy replaced anger and anxiety; he relaxed and his pain diminished. He could hardly believe it. In fact, his old way of thinking was to resist, but if he relaxed, he couldn't miss the basic fact that it was working.

Active Role

CBT encourages you to realize that you must play an active role in your therapy. You must be an involved participant, and it is imperative that you understand that you *can* change the pain. Once you stop believing you are a passive victim in a situation over which you have no control, real changes can and will begin to happen. As demonstrated by Paul and Sam, when they took control over even one episode of debilitating pain, their views were altered, and better still, their pain decreased.

Usually CBT therapists have a specific agenda and structure their sessions to work on specific techniques and concepts. For CBT to be successful, you must be willing to do homework and practice what you have learned during your sessions with the therapist.

One of the most encouraging aspects of CBT is that learning and growing do not stop once treatments with the therapist are finished. You can continue to practice and develop additional coping skills. Researchers have found that even CBT computer programs have been helpful for some clients.

More CBT Benefits

Whether from one-on-one sessions, group therapy, or even computer sessions, CBT has been shown to be beneficial, especially in treating depression, stress, anxiety, or situations that are affected by these conditions, such as chronic pain. CBT can change the way you *think* about pain, which ultimately can change the way you *feel* pain. It also can help you become more active, which is another way to lessen pain.

You can take a more active role in your CBT pain treatment by monitoring your progress. By keeping a written record of the strength of your pain, moods, how much pain medication you are taking, and your activity levels, you can gain insight into how well the CBT treatment is working.

As with any psychoanalytical therapy, there is always a chance that it won't be effective for some people or that problems will return once the active therapy is over. Therapists often schedule return visits, and clients are always encouraged to continue building on their successes.

Phyllis had learned a lot by visiting a therapist she found through her recovery network. This therapist was kind and gentle with Phyllis, never demanding, the way her father had been; nor did the therapist disappear like Phyllis's mother or her many unrequited lovers.

In therapy, Phyllis hunkered down and looked at how she thought about life and her pain. Some of her hot thoughts consisted of negative self-messages like "I'll never change" and "I should go get high; that always worked before, and damn the consequences." She learned in therapy to challenge that way of thinking and to see life more clearly, more as it really was. Her ideas about her pain were tied to her experience with her mother—bedridden and absent and depressed and hopeless. In fact, Phyllis's identity was tied to her mother.

Phyllis's therapist helped her challenge those beliefs. She helped Phyllis see that she was not her mother; in fact, she hadn't spent a day in bed since she got out of the hospital months before. When Phyllis's body ached, she could follow the new path she and her therapist had mapped out in therapy, one filled with hope and positive energy. And, as promised, her pain decreased. It became less significant, kind of an annoyance instead of an all-consuming curse. She started to stand up straighter and look people in the eye and smile and laugh again.

Acceptance and Commitment Therapy (ACT)

Acceptance and commitment therapy finds its roots in **relational frame theory** and utilizes metaphors and experiential exercises. It is based on the principle that we all experience certain emotions, thoughts, memories, and physical sensations that are unpleasant. Problems are caused by trying to avoid or alter the actual experience. This is especially true when resisting or avoiding feelings that arise from the pain, which causes more pain.

ACT believes that "cognitive fusion" of thoughts influences feelings; for example, trying *not* to think of something causes you to think of it more.

ACT promotes mindful awareness of thoughts and feelings—it helps you separate the thought from troublesome feelings associated with it. When Sam was told that he would eventually become crippled because of his scoliosis, rather than become despondent and hopeless about this pronouncement (which was actually wholly inaccurate and untrue), he developed a pattern of associating every ache and pain with the fear and anger that he would be crippled soon. ACT helped him disassociate the pain from those disabling emotions. He learned to continue to function in life effectively, even though the thought that he might be crippled some day was present. This is called **values-consistent behavior**. Sam could accept all the thoughts and feelings associated with his condition but he could separate himself, with practice, from the *meaning* of these thoughts and feelings.

The process of creating values-consistent behaviors starts with identifying what is valuable in your life. Next, what are the reasons to change your thoughts? You can learn to challenge the thoughts and feelings: "I am not crippled now," says Sam; "in fact, I'm going out for a walk. Though I may be crippled some day, I have heard from my physical therapist and two other doctors that most people with scoliosis do not end up in a wheelchair. I don't need to focus on the message of the first surgeon, who was quite misinformed about a lot of things about my condition."

Sam's therapist asked him a critical question: "If you didn't have this pain, how would your life be different?" Sam struggled with this question for weeks, starting with "But I do have this pain and it has ruined my damn life," and ending with finally seeing that the pain had actually enhanced his capacity to feel for others. It actually taught him about compassion. He was able to see the pain as a gift.

Acceptance is a tool that is well known as part of twelve-step programs. It involves surrender rather than a futile attempt to control the uncontrollable (in Buddhist terms, attachment). Studies have shown that these accepting behaviors correlate with less pain intensity, depression, anxiety, and disability, and greater activity and well-being. Sam finally concluded that his pain might not change, so he had to change his life—experience the good and the bad. When he asked himself, "What do you want your life to stand for?" Sam came up with a list that included being of value to others, caring more for others than himself, educating himself and others about scoliosis and chronic pain, and looking forward to dating and making a life with someone.

He developed committed action to move toward the values that he found to be important to him. He started to go to movies; he began to exercise gradually, increasing his core strength with Pilates and sit-ups; and he decided to go back to school with the intention of using his experience with chronic pain to write and teach at the local community college. He volunteered at a local hospital orthopedic ward to work with kids who had spinal problems. He called a woman he had encountered at a workshop a few months before who seemed very interested in him, and they started dating.

ACT also helps you decrease your sense of self as context. In other words, Sam came to realize "I am *not* my struggles or what I am trying to change." He found a distinction between his sense of self and his work with his chronic pain. "I am more than my pain. It is *not* who I am or my identity."

One key factor in ACT is being willing to accept even though pain may not lessen. Sam's new mantra became "I will be okay and my life can have meaning and purpose. This is true value for my life. And today I am not crippled. I'm not so sure I ever will be."

Another technique that is important for ACT is a focus on the present moment, utilizing techniques of mindfulness, which will be discussed next.

Mindfulness

Mindfulness is a set of techniques based on the observation of thoughts and feelings and body sensations without judgment, and on enhancing your conscious awareness of your internal experience. Many of these techniques have been developed over the years from Theraveda and Mahayana Buddhism, which are nonreligious traditions founded around 500 BC. The primary focus is on insight, or *vipassana*. This type of meditation does not seek to eliminate pain or stress, but rather to guide the individual to use intentional, focused, and relaxed awareness to help achieve nonjudgmental self-acceptance in the present moment.

Like tuning an instrument, daily mindfulness practice enriches the brain's neuronal structures, enhances connections, and affects neurotransmitter levels by decreasing cortisol and epinephrine (stimulation) and increasing serotonin and GABA (relaxation). In other words, developing a consistent practice of mindfulness can change the brain.

After years of suffering from chronic pain, you can become attached to it because your pain seems grounding. It is solid and familiar. Attachment to thoughts or outcomes and desiring a different physical state, that is, living without chronic pain, are the cornerstones upon which you expand your suffering. The freedom that mindfulness can offer is that you can change your relationship with your pain and learn to detach from the feelings and physical sensations associated with chronic pain.

> *Mindfulness practice encourages you to be in the moment*
> *without becoming consumed or attached to it.*

Mindfulness practice encourages you to be in the moment without becoming consumed or attached to it. The techniques utilize gentleness toward yourself. I encourage you to be open-hearted to new possibilities that will come from just following your breath. I urge you to let go of the disdain and bitterness you may feel about your pain as you begin to meditate and simply notice what comes up in each moment, changing with each breath that you take.

It will help to work with a teacher or to join a meditation group. Sitting with your pain takes courage, actually more courage than fighting against it. Mindfulness is full of paradoxes; allow it to open you, and open to it. By all means, do what my meditation teacher stressed to me, which is to be kind and loving toward yourself as you work with your breath. There is no "right way" to do this and no goal to achieve.

It is helpful to utilize humor and softness as you attempt to learn to meditate. A good analogy is that this is like training a puppy. The puppy is terribly cute, so when it wanders from the paper, you gently shoo it back—no harsh words for the puppy or for yourself. Just use gentle energy to remind yourself to focus on the breath, and the next breath, and the next after that.

Try not to focus on an outcome; rather, be present for the process. One study found that after three months of daily meditation, those who meditated experienced less pain, improved attention, enhanced well-being, and improved their quality of life. Not too shabby for a process intrinsic in your body, that is, the breath. This breath is available for you any time you like, to work with for free.

Sam joined a meditation group with great reluctance. He had been raised in the confines of a strict religion, and at first the group seemed to have religious overtones. He sat for fifteen minutes, struggling in the beginning with restlessness, anxiety, and increased pain. Over a few weeks' time, he found that his daily practice at home made it easier to sit with the group. Indeed, his mind became less busy, and he was able to sit for longer periods without shifting positions. He looked forward to the group experience because he noted some force beyond just himself that he felt when he was with others who were also sitting quietly. He couldn't identify the day, but it was sometime after a few months of regular attendance and meditating that his pain was imperceptible for longer periods than it was present. He truly felt lucky and blessed for the first time in his life. He couldn't remember when he had felt so good.

This chapter focuses on just these specific techniques to deal with your thoughts and emotions. I encourage you to investigate your local area for groups and therapists who might be able to help guide you in these efforts. Practicing with others is key to learning, changing, and feeling less isolated.

CHAPTER **8**

What Is Pain Recovery?

A Solution to Your Suffering from Chronic Pain

"With the help of the thorn in my foot,
I spring higher than anyone with sound feet."

Søren Kierkegaard

For many of you with chronic pain, traditional pain management approaches and the use of pain medication have not worked, and your pain continues. Many of you have developed an addiction to pain medications and seek alternative options. For those who are not getting positive results from your pain management plan, "pain recovery" is an alternative solution.

Pain recovery is a solution-focused and comprehensive approach to treating chronic pain, encompassing mental, emotional, spiritual, and physical functioning. By balancing these areas and building bridges of mutual support with peers and allies, chronic pain sufferers can learn to accept and live with pain, but let go of suffering.

Pain recovery is about distinguishing between the physical pain and the suffering caused by it, and achieving relief from that suffering. Pain may be inevitable; suffering is not. It occurs in response to thoughts such as "Why me?" or "It isn't fair!" or "I can't stand it!" Suffering helps to cause, and usually results from, feelings of anxiety, anger, fear, depression, frustration, and hopelessness. Pain recovery is a process of learning how to accept pain, while reducing suffering.

Scientific research continually generates evidence of the direct connection between the mind and body. Whatever affects one will inevitably affect the other, regardless of where a problem originates. As a result, imbalances in thinking can cause imbalances in emotional, physical, and spiritual functioning. Pain recovery focuses on restoring that balance. Through this process it is possible to experience decreased pain and improved functioning, without the use of opioid medications.

Pain recovery involves walking a path of continuous learning, growing, and healing. It applies the principles of the Twelve Steps of recovery to the challenges of living with chronic pain. Many recovery programs employ the twelve-step model because it has helped countless numbers of people to recover from a variety of addiction manifestations and compulsive behaviors. The millions of people who have recovered serve as proof that the principles found in these programs are effective.

Pain recovery creates opportunities to consider mental, emotional, spiritual, and physical solutions and strategies to accept chronic pain and learn how to live in peaceful coexistence with it. The goal of pain recovery is to enable those with chronic pain to address their pain in healthier ways and gain freedom from thinking, feeling, and acting like a victim. Through this process, those with chronic pain can learn to live comfortably, with some sense of ease, and free from habit-forming substances.

Pain Management vs. Pain Recovery

The primary goal of pain management is to control, if not eliminate, pain. Pain management involves prescribing pain medications and physical interventions that range from less invasive to more invasive, such as physical therapy, steroid injections, and surgeries. Opioids, or painkillers as they are often called, are the primary medications used to treat chronic pain. They have the potential for significant side effects, along with the possibility of abuse, physical dependence, and addiction.

As discussed in earlier chapters, sometimes using opioids actually causes more pain—a phenomenon known as opioid-induced hyperalgesia. This condition often affects people with chronic pain who are on opioids for long periods of time. The most effective treatment for it is stopping these medications so the brain can "reset" and eliminate the hyperalgesic effect of the opioids.

Obviously, physical interventions like spinal injections, nerve blocks, and other more aggressive treatments have their own risks, some of which are considerable. Chronic pain patients and their caregivers must weigh the level of pain and the potential benefits of what is usually temporary relief against these problematic consequences in the pain management process. With surgery, there are some successes, but many bad outcomes as well.

The goal of eliminating pain altogether from most chronic pain conditions is simply not realistic. The goal of pain recovery is to learn ways to accept and live in coexistence with pain, rather than "kill" it with painkillers.

> *The goal of pain recovery is to learn ways to accept and live in coexistence with pain, rather than "kill" it with painkillers.*

For people with chronic pain, there is a correlation between negative thinking and beliefs and the level of pain they experience. In other words, the more negative the thoughts and beliefs, the greater the pain sensations. This can easily and quickly become a vicious circle, as pain triggers negative thoughts and self-talk, which translate into feelings of suffering as well as increased muscle tension and stress, which in turn amplify the pain signals, triggering more of them. Suffering can be modified because it responds to measures that help a person think differently about his or her pain.

Like any other form of recovery, pain recovery takes time, attention, and energy. Some people may not identify with the term "recovery" because it is commonly associated with addiction. Recovery is basically the process of moving from imbalance to balance. Pain recovery uses the tools of acceptance, hope, an open-minded attitude, and willingness to take positive action. Once you can accept your powerlessness over the existence of chronic pain, you become empowered to assume personal responsibility and can begin the recovery process.

Pain Management vs. Pain Recovery	
Pain Management	**Pain Recovery**
Medically managed	Individually managed
Medication-based	Abstinence-based
Medical model	Twelve-step model
Dependent on medications and medical procedures to "kill" pain	Personal responsibility; learning to accept and coexist with pain
Victim/Patient	Empowered/Advocate
Externally focused	Internally focused
Problem-oriented	Solution-oriented

The Four Points of Balance

Pain recovery is grounded in finding balance (1) physically, (2) mentally, (3) emotionally, and (4) spiritually. This framework creates awareness of the aspects of yourself that, when you are unbalanced, lead to problems in your life. The four points of balance are used to help you identify the areas where imbalance has caused unmanageability in your life and with your family. These points are, of course, interconnected.

Finding recovery requires paying attention to every point and the effect each has on the others. Additionally, your relationships and actions are a reflection of your internal state of balance. Chronic pain is a manifestation of imbalance, typically physical, but also mental, emotional, and spiritual. Developing an awareness of the points and applying the necessary corrections to bring them back into balance is where the solutions to chronic pain and other life challenges lie. As a result of finding balance in pain recovery, your pain levels will diminish.

CHAPTER 9

Families Hurt Too

*"Hurting families look good, but feel bad—
doing their suffering behind closed doors."*

Sharon Wegscheider-Cruse

Chronic pain can be overwhelming. It can destroy every aspect of a person's life. Jobs can be lost, self-esteem disappears, and depression and feelings of worthlessness gradually become the norm. It is not surprising that your suffering with chronic pain affects all those who care about you. Even a once-smoothly operating family can find itself in chaos, with its dynamic inexorably changed by a member in chronic pain.

Families of someone in chronic pain also find they are being affected by something outside their control. They are forced to make adjustments separately and collectively to accommodate both the person in pain and the condition itself. You feel trapped because your loved one has a medical problem and you are helpless to do anything about it.

Before Paul went for treatment, Lila, his wife, felt awful. She didn't know what to do about her miserable life with Paul. She didn't want to leave him. How could she possibly leave him in the throes of addiction and horrible pain? He was, after all, the father of her child, and despite all they had been through, she still loved him, or at least loved who he used to be and who she desperately hoped he could be again.

They fought all the time—about little things and about his deteriorated state. After fighting almost daily, Lila invariably felt guilty. She was so angry, and her anger often came out sideways. She hated to raise her voice in front of the baby. She felt that she should be stronger and be able to help Paul more. They had married for better or worse, and it had really gotten bad. She didn't know if she could hang in there the way her mother would urge her to. Lila saw her mom as a long-suffering martyr who stayed with an abusive, alcoholic husband for thirty-five years until he died of liver failure a few years ago. She'd be damned if she'd repeat that life script and stay with Paul if he didn't get better.

Lila often wondered if he really was in as much pain as he said he was. She couldn't stand being with him when he had taken enough medication to make him "nod out"—head drooping, eyes half-closed, and drooling out of the corner of his mouth. When she would nudge him, he would awake with a jolt and slur out a few words and then nod off again. This was now almost a daily occurrence. When he grimaced with pain as he squirmed away from her touch or if he moved wrong, she felt like her heart was being torn out. She could barely tolerate being around him after a year of this. He was either nodding or complaining, and neither one left her feeling anything but miserable and helpless.

Lila had given up most of her friends, who urged her to come out with them for a lunch or tennis game. She hadn't exercised in months. How could she leave Paul alone? Even if she got a sitter, it would be like taking care of two babies. After all, whoever she asked would have to sit with Paul and make sure he didn't burn the house down with a cigarette, or God knows what else might happen. It made her so mad, and she felt frustrated and miserable and trapped.

"I Feel Your Pain . . ."

When people have chronic pain, they usually can give a name to the sensations they are having. They may say their pain is burning, throbbing, aching, sharp, dull, fiery, heavy, slight, pins and needles, fleeting, long-lasting, or tingling, and on and on. Although family members, as observers, don't actually feel what the person in pain is feeling, much of the time they understand what's going on based on their own personal experiences of pain. And this is true everywhere, with everyone.

Whether you know the person in pain or not, as a caring person you often sympathize with him or her. That is, you can understand and appreciate that this person has pain. "Oh, you poor thing," you might say.

Recent studies have revealed, however, that the human reaction to someone else's pain is light-years beyond mere sympathy or simply understanding that someone else is in pain. While you don't actually feel another person's sensation of pain, when you see someone in pain your brain reacts almost as though it's you who is experiencing the pain. Clinical tests show that true understanding of another's pain draws on brain circuits in the somatosensory cortex that "mirror" those the person is using as he or she feels pain. In other words, when you watch someone undergo something painful, your brain "lights up" in the same areas where the brain of the person in pain is lighting up.

While you don't actually feel another person's sensation of pain, when you see someone in pain your brain reacts almost as though it's you who is experiencing the pain.

Lila's reaction to Paul's pain was natural. She couldn't help herself, as the studies show. She really did "feel" Paul's pain.

Furthermore, these studies reveal that you don't even have to see the actual occurrence of the painful experience for your brain to react. All you have to do is see a person act as if he or she is in pain, and your brain lights up. This "empathetic" reaction has been proven by researchers who took functional magnetic resonance imaging (fMRI) scans of a person's brain when shown videos of the face of another person who was in pain. There is an amazing overlap in the areas of the brain that are set in motion when you undergo pain and the areas of the brain that activate when you see someone else in the midst of pain.

While the experience of pain is individual, expressions of pain, such as furrowing your brow, frowning, or squinting, have an obvious survival and communicative value. Facial expressions of pain can warn others of dangerous situations and elicit helping behavior. The fMRI studies also show that not only is the pain shared, but the intensity of the observed pain becomes encoded in the observer's brain. Seeing another person experience pain causes responses in the part of your brain responsible for producing emotional reactions to the physical sensations of pain.

These studies show that it's part of being human to react empathetically to someone in pain. It's wired into our brains. Actually, this is part of a built-in social instinct that we all have. We watch out for others in our "herd," which leads to better survival for all of us. "I feel your pain" is almost an undeniable truism. And it is only natural to infer that when the person you see in pain is someone in your own family, someone you care deeply about, your reaction to his or her pain is exponentially stronger. Empathy for a loved family member in chronic pain is not something you can turn on or off. When you love the person in pain, you want to do whatever you can to help stop the pain, or at least make it as bearable as possible.

Family "Organism"

The family is a complex organism. And, like any organism or system that has diverse parts that make up the whole, it functions best when all the different elements are in good working order. Often, the system can completely break down when one part becomes broken or dysfunctional.

Systems theory is an interdisciplinary field, the study of the nature of complex systems in nature, society, and science. By using the theory, it is possible to analyze and describe any group of objects that work in concert to produce a result. The family has been identified as such a system.

Each member of a healthy family takes part in the dynamic functions of the family, where each has responsibilities and roles to play. Additionally, there is support within a healthy family that encourages each member to act independently.

Family systems research has developed an understanding of the family as an organism. Families are more than just individuals who live together. Everything that happens to one member has an effect on others within the family system. Therefore, if one member is in pain, the equilibrium of the family shifts and each family member changes and adjusts accordingly. After a while, the symptoms seem to take on a life of their own and seem necessary for the family to function, even if the symptoms aren't needed.

This strain of one of its members in pain is a struggle even in a well-functioning family. Mom in pain does not parent the way she used to; an adult son in pain becomes dependent on his parents while they are preparing for retirement, not parenthood; a spouse in pain may no longer provide emotional, financial, or sexual support.

Family system theory works with families as they exist by trying to coordinate the strengths of each member into the reality of a painful condition for one of its members.

Setting up flexible roles for each member is vital for families. Roles are patterns of behavior by which individuals fulfill functions and needs within the family. When role responsibilities are taken seriously, most families can usually cope not only with the stresses and strains of everyday life, but also with unexpected crises and normal changes that occur over time.

Family roles include parent, spouse, aunt, brother, sister, child, grandparent, and so on. Connected with each role are specific expectations within the family on how those roles should be performed. Healthy families are expected to provide money, food, shelter, and clothing for all members; to be nurturing and supportive of other members, including providing warmth, comfort, and reassurance; to provide life skills development for both children and adults; to maintain and manage the family system, including discipline and enforcement of behavioral standards; and, in a marriage, to provide for the sexual needs of both partners.

In a healthy family, roles are clearly identifiable so that everyone knows what his or her responsibilities are. Ideally, these roles should be allocated fairly so all family members feel they are doing their part and the family unit is running smoothly and responsibly.

Obviously, when someone in a family is injured, it will have an impact on everyone in that family. When dad breaks his leg, the entire family is forced to change and make allowances for the situation. However, when the calamity is long-term, such as in the case of chronic pain, it becomes more than merely making allowances for the situation. Everyone's life changes.

These changes can be social, economic, physical, and psychological. In most cases, family members at first draw together while readily accepting other roles and responsibilities. However, as the situation continues for months or even years, the family can begin to experience considerable stress and changes are bound to occur.

Sam had returned home to live with his parent and younger siblings after his last surgery. He could no longer manage cooking, cleaning, and maintaining an apartment on his own. As days stretched into weeks, his mom, Eleanor, became weary of the added responsibilities of shopping for the right organic products that Sam demanded. Frank, his dad, missed more golf games than he cared to admit, and when he did get to go, he was cranky and preoccupied to the point where he decided not to play until this situation with Sam was resolved. But how on Earth was that going to happen? Sam seemed to be getting worse, not better, and Frank grew more and more frustrated with the lack of a plan to get Sam better and out of the house.

Sam's younger brother, Joey, was devastated. He had to share a room with Sam, who dominated the landscape with his booming voice and demanding ways. Joey found his privacy compromised and became depressed. Alicia, who was just twelve years old, idolized her big brother Sam, and couldn't come to terms with him using a cane and being drugged a good part of the time. She withdrew from the family, spending more time with friends and returning home only to eat and sleep.

Frank and Eleanor found themselves arguing about how to address the worsening situation with Sam. "We can't kick him out, Frank! Where would he go?" Eleanor looked at her husband with consternation and misery. He hated to see her this way, and had to admit that he had no finite suggestions for how their now-disabled son, who had become dependent on strong medications, could possibly function without their assistance. They had little time to attend to the growing dysfunction in the lives of their adolescent children, Joey and Alicia. Like Lila, Eleanor and Frank felt helpless and trapped.

Dr. Hanson describes some common family problems that can result from long-term chronic pain. They include:

- Withdrawal from normal family activities. Many people isolate themselves from the rest of the family when they're in pain. Some shun family activities and outings.

- Alienating your family as a result of irritability and temper outbursts. It's a sad fact that many in chronic pain take their frustrations out on the people closest to them. If your pain makes you irritable and frustrated, you can alienate family members through crankiness and losing your temper. Your actions can compound your already delicate problem by adding guilt for your actions. It puts added stress on the family because they may feel like they have to continually "walk on eggshells" to avoid further upsets.

- Losing identity. Chronic pain can hinder activities that once supported your feelings of masculinity or femininity. Some women believe they are less than a woman if they are unable to do activities associated with the female role such as cooking, cleaning, and child care. Men may feel they are less than a man if they aren't doing the roles traditionally assigned to men like bringing home a paycheck or playing sports with the kids. Chronic pain can cause a complete role reversal. Additionally, chronic pain can interfere with a person's sexual identity by making him or her unable to enjoy relations with his or her mate.

- Being treated like an invalid. Family members can treat someone in chronic pain as though they're more helpless than they really are. The family may be more protective than necessary.

- Being misunderstood. On the other side of the coin, some families have a difficult time grasping how bad off a family member in chronic pain can be. A common complaint is that the family expects more than the person in pain is actually capable of doing.

The real key to maintaining health as a family system is being able to adapt to changing circumstances. In general systems theory (GST), a system that is unyielding and unable to change is considered a sick system. Ludwig Von Bertlanffy was an early pioneer in GST and his works are an integral part of understanding how systems work and why they break down.

Therefore, as chronic pain takes over someone in the family system, it is often necessary for each member to reorganize and to acknowledge and accept different roles and responsibilities in order to maintain the healthy family.

New or altered roles are likely to be long-term, but changing, so it is necessary for the family to reassess the situation on a regular basis and be flexible. The reassessment will help the person in pain understand that he or she has not lost total control of his or her life and that he or she can grow and change, and so can the family. Understanding that the whole family is being affected gives everyone involved an opportunity to identify and take care of potential problems.

Helping Families

Many family troubles linked to chronic pain can be addressed by being open and honest. Problems generally develop over time and only escalate because members try to avoid acknowledging them. Communication is a two-way street and involves not only expressing what you are feeling and getting others in the family to see your point of view, but also listening to others and really trying to understand what they are experiencing.

Ideally, when a member is in chronic pain, the family adjusts and continues life as a cohesive, successfully functioning unit. Unfortunately, however, this is often not the case. In many cases of chronic pain, the family makes changes, but then reality sets in. The family member in pain doesn't get better. Life drags on, and "burnout" becomes as threatening as the painful condition.

Dr. Hanson describes three ways in which family members respond to expressions of pain:

1   *Punishing responses.* Family members may ignore you or respond in ways that indicate a lack of care or concern, including irritation, frustration, or anger.

2   *Solicitous responses.* Family members become extremely helpful (often too much so), getting your medicine, getting your food or water, or taking over your chores.

3   *Distracting responses.* Your family tries to distract you from your pain. Members encourage you to do things like read, work on a hobby, or move around.

Of these three, punishing responses are the least desirable. Minimizing or disregarding the painful situation can make a person's emotional condition all the worse. Responding with anger, resentment, or frustration can have a ruinous effect on a relationship, as it did with Lila and Paul.

Concern and compassion are healthy, but solicitous responses may be overdone and actually reinforce helplessness. Experimental studies have found that the presence of a solicitous spouse increased pain intensity and more than doubled brain activity from an electrical shock administered to a patient with chronic pain. This shows that being rewarded for experiencing pain (receiving increased attention, for example) can increase the amount of pain one experiences.

It is natural for someone in pain to occasionally react to his or her condition with a moan or groan, but some in chronic pain are continually calling attention to their condition. When this happens, the solicitous spouse (or child or parent) may find he or she is reacting not to the painful condition, but to the moan. The mate who consistently responds to the moans and groans is actually reinforcing the pain. The same principle applies to people in chronic pain who stand to gain from their pain disability. Receiving benefits for having pain can make the pain more intense and frequent. It is important to realize that these processes do not involve conscious exaggeration or deceit. They are simply learned responses from receiving a reward (attention, service, or money) for being in pain. It's as simple as that. Conversely, rewarding function increases function.

There is a fine line between compassion and codependence. Compassion is unconditional kindness for oneself and others. It is the healthy understanding that "I'm okay, and I care about you and want you and others to be okay, too." Compassion is universal and based in the individual's willingness to be caring, but not at his or her own expense. Codependency differs from compassion in that it develops from a need for the well-being of others. Codependency generates from an inner feeling of deficiency. "I can't be okay if you are not okay."

One of the fundamental differences between compassion and codependency is in the ability for self-care. Compassionate people are gentle with themselves, so that they may better care for another. Codependent people lose sight of their needs in the needs of another.

Eleanor was an inveterate codependent. She was totally devoted to Frank and their children and would neglect her own needs in order to take care of them. After years of marriage, they had come to an understanding of each other's styles and needs, and some balance was achieved. Eleanor had her own hobbies and activities outside the home, and she and Frank both enjoyed their time together as well. The kids had their lives full of sports, studies, and friends and were growing up well. Frank liked having meals prepared, but had grown used to preparing dinner for himself, Joey, and Alicia every other Tuesday when Eleanor was volunteering at the local hospital. She'd always bring home dessert, and it made their family time together feel more valuable.

When Sam came to live with them, everything changed. Eleanor developed a desperate need to control his environment and, though it was futile, his pain. She bought him a new mattress, cooked whatever exotic thing he was in the mood for, put up with unending and unreasonable demands for comfort enhancers, and demanded nothing in return. And as she became more enmeshed with Sam, she provided less and less support to her husband and other children.

Distracting responses are of the greatest benefit to those in pain, as well as to their family members. As discussed in other areas in this book, doing some type of activity, even if it's as slight as getting your own drink of water, is one of the best things you can do for yourself when you're in pain. And the family that encourages any kind of activity that reinforces independence is helping the person in pain.

Dr. Julie K. Silver, in her book *Chronic Pain and the Family: A New Guide*, describes beneficial ways in which the person in pain and family members can reduce or eliminate maladaptive chronic pain behaviors. The person in pain should:

- "Use words to describe what you're experiencing. Keep in mind, though, that people don't need to hear exactly how you're feeling. There are many times when 'suffering in silence' will be beneficial to you and your family members.

- Don't hold your spouse or other loved ones responsible for your physical comfort. If you need something and can get it yourself, then do so.

- Try to avoid canceling plans with people—it's disappointing for them and for you. If you can manage the activity, then go ahead and do it.

- Understand that the less active you are, the more pain you'll have as a result of physical deconditioning. So try to remain as active as possible.

- If you're unable to handle household responsibilities that were once yours, then take on new ones that you can manage in order to lessen the burden on your loved ones.

- Be your own advocate and seek legitimate medical treatment. Follow your doctor's advice unless there is a compelling reason not to. If you don't want to do something your doctor recommends, then discuss this with him so that an alternate treatment plan can be implemented.

- Engage in regular, but not incessant, honest and open communication with your family members about what's happening to you and how you're feeling. Ask them how they're feeling and listen with empathy. Remember that just because you're feeling the physical pain doesn't mean they're not suffering as well."

Family members:

- "Don't constantly ask how your loved one is feeling—particularly when the person is not complaining or focusing on the pain.

- Encourage the person in pain to do whatever he can to help himself and the family.

- Avoid taking over all the responsibilities of the family—ask and expect the person in pain to help whenever possible.

- Don't be the go-between for the person in pain and the doctor—they should have their own relationship, and the person in pain should be responsible for following through with all treatment plans.

- Don't cancel your plans to do things just because someone else is in pain. Enjoy the things that you can do. Keep in mind that children often cope the same way their parents do. If your children see you shut down and become reclusive, they may do the same. On the other hand, if they see you enjoying yourself and having fun despite difficulties at home, they will likely respond in kind.

- Engage in honest and loving communication on a regular basis with both the person in pain and other members of the family who may be affected as well.

- Don't respond to maladaptive pain behaviors. If you can, point out these behaviors in a loving way and try to reinforce the fact that they're not useful."

Phyllis and her Aunt Ellie made a good team. Aunt Ellie was a veteran of "tough love" experiences, having lost two teenaged children to the ravages of drug abuse. Now that she had a chance with her niece, she was applying all of the healthy skills she had learned by going to Nar-Anon meetings.

She was loving and compassionate and consistent and firm. "I'm sorry you're sore today, dear. Now get up and wash your face; we're going for our morning walk. See you in ten minutes downstairs." She was cheerful and even-tempered, and Phyllis responded. After all, Phyllis knew she always felt better after their walks.

Aunt Ellie accompanied Phyllis to yoga class and enjoyed their time together. She also had a rich, full life of her own and was diligent in maintaining her activities. Her positive disposition served her and Phyllis well—and both thrived in their household.

Healthy families take care of themselves—each individual enhances the family and does not become lost in the chronic pain of one of its members.

CHAPTER **10**

Treatment Modalities

"Success is dependent on effort."

Sophocles

More than anything else, those in chronic pain want to stop the hurt. For most, it may become more important than food or sleep, often because pain is a primary obstacle to eating or sleeping. There are many strategies used to help people cope with debilitating pain. These include the more general treatment methods such as physical therapy, medications that range from the mild to the strong, and surgery. Since chronic pain has no single cause or enabling feature, treatment methods are extremely varied.

As I wrote this book, I found this chapter to be the longest. This is a positive sign, since it means there are many, many choices for you to take advantage of to decrease your pain and suffering. I suggest you sample a number of different techniques to see if any are helpful. Unlike taking a pill, these methods take time until you see and feel an effect. You will need to repeat any of these techniques a number of times regularly (at least for a month or two) before you may see an improvement in how you feel. Some things work for some people some of the time. Keep in mind that just because a therapy or treatment works for one person doesn't mean it will work for you. After a while, you may find some of these treatments stop working. There is always a need to monitor the effect and modify the plan accordingly if the effect is lost.

I suggest you keep track of pain scores before and after trying any of these methods and track changes daily, weekly, and monthly to see if they are helping. One simple way to do this is to "grade" your pain on a one-to-ten scale, with one being little or no pain and ten being the worst pain you've ever felt. Some people feel so bad that they report their pain to be at a fifteen, but for the purposes of consistency, it helps to stick to this scale of grading.

The following is the best pain scale I've seen to describe severity, though not necessarily quality, of pain. Remember, whenever a doctor asks you to rate your pain from one to ten, ask for a pain scale so you can be sure you are both speaking the same language.

PAIN SCALE

0—Pain-free.

1—Very minor annoyance; occasional minor twinges.

2—Minor annoyance; occasional strong twinges.

3—Annoying enough to be distracting.

4—Can be ignored if you are really involved in your work, but still distracting.

5—Can't be ignored for more than thirty minutes.

6—Can't be ignored for any length of time, but you can still go to work and participate in social activities.

7—Makes it difficult to concentrate; interferes with sleep. You can still function with effort.

8—Physical activity severely limited. You can read and converse with effort. Nausea and dizziness set in as factors of pain.

9—Unable to speak. Crying out or moaning uncontrollably; near delirium.

10—Unconscious. Pain makes you pass out.

You may find that a pill might reduce pain from an eight to a three, but that change might only last fifteen to twenty minutes and leave you feeling "doped up." These techniques might cause smaller and less noticeable improvement, perhaps from a seven to a five, but the effects increase over time. If something works once, it is only logical that it will work again if you keep at it. Practice will enhance the benefits. Also, it is totally appropriate and recommended to combine many techniques that seem helpful to you. So stick with it.

Phyllis was on a roll. She emerged from thirty days of treatment following detox with a good handle on her addiction and pain. She was drug-free for the first time in years and had a positive and hopeful attitude that she hadn't felt in quite a while. She went to yoga class twice a week and did her favorite stretching poses several times a day. She felt energized and fulfilled, especially after the relaxation part of the class. She loved the feeling of exploring her "edges" without pushing beyond her means.

The acupuncturist Phyllis worked with in treatment was available to her weekly through her insurance, so she set up a regular schedule. The needle treatments left her muscles less sore and also gave her some energy. She slept better, especially when she listened to the **body scan** tapes prepared for her in treatment. After years of inactivity, Phyllis joined the gym, walked on the treadmill, and occasionally attended a Pilates class. She began feeling stronger and more in control of her pain. The better she felt, the more committed to continuing all her healthy activities she became. And best of all, her pain was lower than it had been on pain pills.

Complementary and Alternative Treatments

Complementary and alternative drugless therapies have been used for thousands of years to treat chronic pain as well as everyday illnesses. "Alternative" means they are out of the mainstream and not always accepted by all conventional medical practitioners. "Complementary" refers to the fact that these treatments are added to other useful therapies. For example, Ayurveda is the traditional medicine of India and has been used for more than 5,000 years in Eastern cultures. It is based on a theory that seeks to integrate and balance the mind, body, and spirit.

Ayurveda means the science of life, and it seeks to create a balance that leads to contentment, health, and prevention of illness—in essence, a wellness program.

Chronic pain is influenced by psychological and social factors in addition to biological aspects, and some of these ancient therapies emphasize the whole person in a holistic approach. Professionals are beginning to understand, prescribe, and use treatment regimens that were once considered out of the ordinary. Several of these are called **complementary and alternative medicine (CAM)** treatments. Some CAMs I will discuss are acupuncture, exercise, aromatherapy, foods and nutrition, oxygen therapy, yoga, reiki, hypnotherapy, hydrotherapy, music therapy, meditation, biofeedback, and chiropractic therapy. These natural forms of therapy are designed to help diminish pain and illness naturally and allow you to be more in control of your life.

After weaning off his medications, Sam felt sore all over a good part of the time. He had lain in bed while his mother, Eleanor, catered to his every demand until she finally put her foot down. "You either start taking care of yourself or you'll have to find somewhere else to live," she said forcefully. He was perplexed by her manner; she was calm and firm. Had someone been training her? Sam wondered. But her calmness got through to the part of him that wanted things—and his life—to be different.

Regardless of where she learned this (he later found out that she had been going to twelve-step meetings and therapy), Sam responded with a sense of obligation and interest. He wanted to be out of bed and return to the world, so he started setting the alarm and going to the gym daily. His dad drove him and helped him around at first, but the more he moved, the more Sam found himself able to do. And unlike in previous attempts to exercise, he hired a trainer who had extensive experience with scoliosis patients, and the trainer worked with Sam on stretching, strengthening, and walking daily. The Jacuzzi and pool ended up being excellent adjuncts to the rest of his workout and offered gentle healing for his sore muscles.

For the first time, Sam was pacing himself. He walked at low speeds on a flat treadmill, and he gradually increased the duration, speed, and incline, with direction from the trainer. He went to a Pilates class with his trainer and learned new breathing exercises in a yoga class he started attending on Fridays at the gym. He resisted the desire to contort his body as he saw the instructor do, settling for the wonderful sense of stretching to his edge, retreating, and pushing just a bit further before releasing the pose and resting. He even allowed himself to sit.

He began to get stronger; the pain was less threatening, and actually less noticeable. It was always there, but it didn't overwhelm Sam, and he improved even more.

Soaking in a hot tub (hydrotherapy) eased aching muscles that seemed to tense up at the slightest provocation. Ice packs and lying on a heating pad also helped. Twenty minutes of the frigid ice often took care of surface muscles, while the hot pad often calmed the deeper tightness of his newly used muscles.

Sam found that gentle stretching before walking loosened his legs and back, quieting the pain and making his walks more effective and enjoyable. As silly as it once sounded to Sam, he found that quietly listening to soothing music helped his pain and helped him cope without getting angry or frustrated.

Today Sam walks three miles every day. He's not ready to run a marathon, nor will he ever be. But he's still drug-free. Every day, too, he has pain, but it does not attack him the way it once did. Sam doesn't know the exact names for his treatments, but his ability to live and function with his pain is based pretty much on several types of complementary and alternative medicines described in this chapter, including exercise, hydrotherapy, physical therapy, music therapy, and others. They helped Sam; maybe they can help you, too.

> *One of the more appealing factors of these types of treatments is that they are not independent of one another; they can be used together.*

One of the more appealing factors of these types of treatments is that they are not independent of one another; they can be used together. One word of caution: Because some of these methods are controversial, it is important that you research and find a good practitioner who is competent and licensed. Don't be afraid to ask questions about the therapy you want to try, as well as where the practitioner studied. It is also a good idea to ask someone who has worked with a practitioner you are considering using. Remember, this is your body and you are responsible for protecting it.

EXERCISE

One of the primary problems with chronic pain is lack of movement—you try to protect yourself from pain and "splint" the places that hurt. Unfortunately, the less you move, the more pain you have when you do move, causing you to move less. It becomes a vicious and painful cycle. The only solution for this chronic "un-movement syndrome" is moving.

Studies have shown that regular and sustained physical activity is beneficial to virtually every system in the body. Exercise, including water exercise, weight training, walking, and aerobic workouts, stimulates the production of endorphins and is very effective in aiding flexibility, mobility, and specific movements, and it actually improves function. Endorphins also help ease anxiety and depression, major components of chronic pain. When you are inactive your body becomes deconditioned, which can add substantially to your perception and experience of pain. Research in which people in chronic pain rode an exercise bicycle for thirty minutes proved that people in chronic pain can substantially reduce their pain by such exercise.

Additionally, exercise can:

- Help you maintain a healthy weight. Dropping extra pounds can lessen the stress you place on your joints, one way to ease bone pain.

- Increase flexibility. As your body gains flexibility, you are less likely to strain, which can add substantially to chronic pain.

- Help you build strength. The stronger you are, the better your muscles can take the load off joints and bones. The healthier the muscle, the less pain you feel.

- Increase serotonin level. Serotonin improves your mood and fights pain by blocking the perception of pain in the brain. It is a natural sleep regulator, and sleep also helps you fight the perception of pain.

- Protect and strengthen the heart and circulatory system. Exercise helps decrease the risk of stroke, heart attack, and diabetes. It also reduces high blood pressure.

- Increase dopamine levels, resulting in improved moods and increased energy. Regular exercise can boost your dopamine levels and add to all the systems your body needs and uses to fight chronic pain.

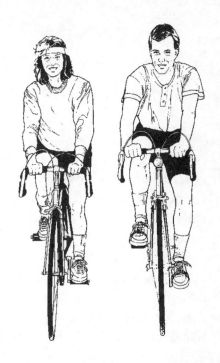

Although the best pain-relieving power of exercise seems to come from sustained aerobic activity like brisk walking, jogging, or riding an exercise bike for thirty minutes or more, any exercise or activity is better than none. Once an exercise program is started, no matter how small or mild, it can be built upon and increased. No one is exactly sure why exercise works as well as it does to relieve pain, but research suggests that exercise retrains the nervous system to build new brain pathways that bypass those hung up on pain signals (refer back to my discussion on the plastic brain).

If you plan to begin an exercise program, you are advised always to consult with your health practitioner first. This is especially true if you are in pain, because it is crucial that the exercises be designed to help alleviate your problems and not increase them by causing injury.

FOODS AND NUTRITION

What we eat every day has a profound effect on how we feel. Our foods play a major role in our health and well-being. Scientists and researchers have concluded that a poor diet contributes to a third of all cancers. According to Dr. Neal Barnard, author of *Foods That Fight Pain*, foods fight pain in four distinct ways:

- They can reduce damage at the site of an injury.

- They work inside the brain to reduce pain sensitivity.

- They act as painkillers on nerves.

- They help our bodies fight inflammation.

Actually, you have been programmed from the time you could walk to use food to ease your pain. Recall that as a child, when you received a minor injury, your parents might have soothed your scraped knee with a treat. In later years, whether it's an active memory or not, your brain recalls how that treat helped your "boo-boos." And who can forget ice cream after you had your tonsils taken out?

More realistically, there is scant evidence that a simple diet change can drive out your chronic pain. However, there is ample evidence that a healthy diet ultimately adds to the length of your life, and being and feeling healthy helps fight pain sensations. It is also important to understand that a good diet can help fight many chronic diseases that often lead to chronic pain or make it worse.

Phyllis had a back condition in addition to her fibromyalgia, but smoking and eating fatty "junk" food only made her pain increase. Also, being overweight put a greater strain on her aching body. Phyllis had put on forty pounds when she stopped using speed and cocaine. She had been cautioned by her doctor to eat wholesome foods such as green

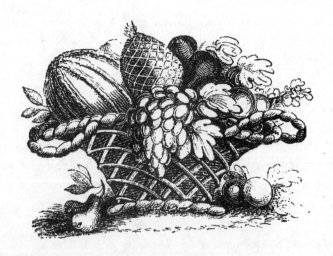

leafy vegetables, whole grains, and fish; however, she would justify eating "junk" food because her pain caused her to feel too tired to cook the good foods she knew she should eat. She became caught in the cycle that many people with chronic pain find themselves in—taking shortcuts because her pain was debilitating, but the shortcuts actually caused more problems. It is not an easy reality to face, but just as your chronic pain did not develop overnight, neither will the solution to finding relief develop in a day or two.

At her gym, Phyllis met with a nutritionist who helped her craft a healthy diet that provided adequate calories while allowing her to lose half a pound every week or two. You can find relief from your pain by incorporating a number of healthy foods into your regular diet, as Phyllis eventually learned. There are even foods that fight swelling and inflammation, and therefore can contribute to pain reduction, for example:

- Tart cherries contain powerful cancer-fighting antioxidants as well as cyanidin, a substance that fights inflammation better than aspirin. Research shows that cherries may also help ease the pain of gout and arthritis.

- Omega-3 fatty acids from fish fight inflammation, as well as heart disease and cholesterol. Studies have shown that participants with rheumatoid arthritis who took omega-3 were able to decrease the amount of nonsteroidal anti-inflammatory drugs (NSAIDs) they took on a regular basis.

- High-protein soybeans are loaded with powerful compounds that slow oxidation and inflammation.

- Turmeric contains curcumin, a substance that has been used in Asia for centuries to fight illness. Modern research shows that the compound fights cancer and inflammation.

- Vitamin D deficiency has been shown to be associated with chronic pain. Supplements may decrease pain levels.

More and more people have found that using herbal painkillers has fewer side effects and long-term risks than traditional medicines.

Additionally, there is no threat of chemical dependency. Research has shown that some herbal medicines not only help relieve pain, but also can attack some of the underlying causes of the pain. One of the most common herbal medicines is white willow bark. It has been used for centuries to relieve pain. It can help reduce acute or chronic pain in the back, joints, teeth, and head.

Other herbs used to fight pain include feverfew, ginger, cat's claw, cayenne, eucalyptus, aloe vera, lobelia, neem, yellow dock, passion flower, hops, and wood betony.

Herbs technically are drugs and should be treated as such. Some can produce side effects and carry risks when not taken responsibly. It is always important to consult with your doctor and pharmacist before taking any herbal preparations since they can have potential reactions with your other medications. Make sure you read labels for warnings and ingredients.

MEDITATION

Meditation is one of the most popular of alternative methods of pain relief. Practitioners say that when people meditate, they can increase the amount of natural painkillers in their body and stimulate the production of pleasurable chemicals. Meditation can encourage a sense of well-being, happiness, connectedness, and wholeness.

Common practices in meditation include:

- Breathing. Practitioners become aware of their breath and how they can control it. Slowing breathing helps to calm the mind. Focus on the breath as the "object of meditation." It helps to slow the heart, lower the blood pressure, and often decrease the pain.

- Transforming the view of life. Meditating helps practitioners alter their view of themselves. Instead of feeling helpless and out of control, you can get a sense of the possible, a self-induced calmness with inner peace and harmony. As your view of yourself changes, you also can create greater balance in your life.

- Visualization. This is a commonly used technique to help with relaxation. You simply visualize a place or activity that brought happiness into your life. This technique often can be facilitated— a guided visualization.

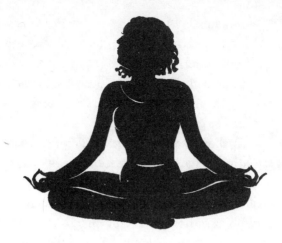

Any meditative techniques can be done alone and in silence, or with an audio track in the background, or in groups, which can be very powerful, and often with the verbal guidance of a teacher.

One specific meditative practice is called the body scan, which is adapted from an ancient Burmese practice used by many practitioners, including Jon Kabat-Zinn, Ph.D., an internationally known scientist and meditation teacher. This guided meditation encourages you to scan through your body much like a CT scan machine might. It utilizes the breath to affect and decrease tension and pain. Each time you encounter these feelings you can replace them with a sense of spaciousness, relaxation, and freedom.

CHIROPRACTIC THERAPY

Chiropractic therapy diagnoses and treats problems involving nerves, bones, muscles, and joints. Chiropractors believe that manipulation of muscles, the spine, and other joints helps the body heal itself. Based on treatments used for thousands of years, chiropractic medicine was founded by Daniel David Palmer in 1895. Palmer reportedly cured a man of deafness and acute back pain by realigning a displaced vertebra in his back. Chiropractic medicine is the third-largest health profession in the Western world. More than 30 million people are treated each year.

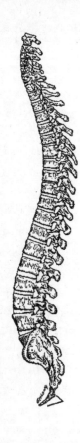

Manipulation is the primary treatment offered by chiropractors, although there are other therapies offered including massage and prescribed exercises. Chiropractors sometimes use various tests to help with their diagnoses, such as x-rays, blood tests, and blood pressure readings.

Although chiropractic medicine has a lot in common with other health professions, it is unique in its belief that spinal misalignment is the cause of most forms of illness. Many people visit a chiropractor for a specific problem; however, chiropractors report that their manipulations benefit the person's health in a general way. There are hundreds of different techniques and methods of manipulation used by chiropractors to treat as many conditions. Research has shown that chiropractic medicine is effective in many cases to reduce and treat acute and chronic back pain. It also has been shown to help many painful conditions including frozen shoulder, muscle spasms, and carpal tunnel syndrome, among others.

PHYSICAL THERAPY

Physical therapy (PT) is the treatment, prevention, and management of movement disorders arising from conditions and diseases. It has its origins in ancient history and was first reported 5,000 years ago in China as massage and manual therapy. Hippocrates explained massage and hydrotherapy in 460 BC. Ayurveda therapists, practitioners of the oldest medical modality known, used PT to manipulate patients' bodies.

Modern PT was started in 1896 to help patients maintain adequate muscle function and mobility. The need to rehabilitate amputees during World War I and World War II, as well as to work with patients suffering from debilitating diseases such as polio, helped make PT a necessary part of twentieth-century medicine. Practitioners believe functional movement is the basis for being healthy.

PT encompasses techniques that include manipulation, traction, massage, therapeutic exercise, functional training, patient education, and counseling about movement and healthy body mechanics. Physical therapists also use ice, heat, electrical currents, and a variety of newer techniques to relieve adhesions (Graston, **active release**) and to decrease sympathetic tone (PRRT). PT involves treatment, healing, and prevention of injuries or disabilities. PT promotes healing, restores function and movement, and relieves pain. Because each individual is different, physical therapists design programs specifically for each person. For example, if you have a sore back because of weak muscles, the therapist will teach you how to strengthen those muscles.

Often pain can be treated with physical therapy through passive and active therapies. Forms of passive therapy include traction, electrical stimulation, ultrasound, hot packs, and ice packs. Active therapy includes aerobic conditioning, strengthening exercises, muscular release, and stretching. Manual therapy is an especially effective method of treating pain. Manual therapy involves restoring movement to stiff joints and reducing muscle tension in order to return a patient to full mobility.

Therapists treat many different diseases and conditions, including:

- Neck and back pain.

- Spinal and joint conditions and pain from arthritis.

- Cerebral palsy and spina bifida.

- Heart and lung conditions.

- Neurological conditions.

- Muscle control and biomechanical conditions.

The main principle that Paul had to perfect was "pacing." He had been an athlete before his accident and wanted to return to pre-accident function now that he was back among the living. His therapist was constantly reminding him

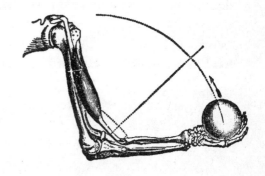

to slow down, breathe, stretch adequately before and after exercising, and, hardest of all, to quit when he was at his edge. He'd been down so long, he couldn't tell clearly when it was time and when he was "wimping out." He worked diligently with his physical and psychological therapist on these very issues. His hard-driving nature served to get him going, but it was through restraint and accepting the limitations of his damaged body that he was able to sustain a program of gradual improvement with results that were paying off.

STRETCHING

Stretching exercises are used to help keep muscles and ligaments limber and flexible. Stretching can ease stiffness, increase your range of movement, reduce stress on joints, and increase the flow of blood and nutrients throughout the body, all of which can help you fight pain. Stretching, or flexibility training, is a way to reduce injuries and increase joint mobility.

As you age, your muscles begin to tighten, lessening your range of motion. You find it's more difficult to do the things you once found easy, such as picking up something from the floor, reaching for something over your head, turning your head while making a U-turn, or even getting dressed in the morning. Stretching helps lengthen your muscles and makes these everyday tasks easier.

The muscles of those of you in chronic pain behave in the same way as in someone getting older, but at a greatly accelerated rate. Pain causes you to use your muscles less and move less, which eventually makes it that much more painful to do just about everything. When you limit the use of your muscles because of pain, they become tighter, which causes more pain. Here are a few examples of what stretching can help accomplish:

- Reduce muscle tension.

- Increase range of movement.

- Improve posture.

- Boost energy.

- Increase strength.

- Increase blood flow.

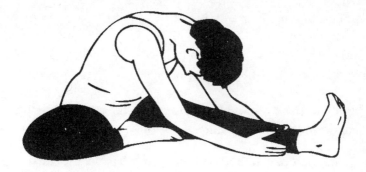

Stretching works by allowing you to decrease resistance.

Phyllis both loved and hated her stretching class. By working with her body, and with the help of an instructor who took a shine to her, Phyllis was able to go to the edge of her perceived limit and breathe, relax, and stretch more. She found a lot of her ability to stretch was limited by her fear that it would hurt. Of course it did hurt, but as she developed trust in her instructor, Phyllis allowed him to coax her limbs into surprising positions. And as she practiced stretching daily, she found her flexibility increased and her pain decreased.

PILATES

Pilates is an innovative system of mind-body exercise developed by Joseph Pilates in the early 1900s. It was designed to build strength without adding bulk and to create a sleek, toned body. The Pilates method, as well as the specially designed apparatus used with the exercises, focuses on core postural muscles that keep the body balanced and are essential to support the spine. Pilates teaches awareness of neutral spine alignment and strengthens the muscles that support this alignment. The alignment helps treat and prevent back pain. It also improves strength, flexibility, and conditioning of the muscles of the hip and pelvic girdle.

Controlled Pilates exercises are performed slowly and gently, while always maintaining good posture. These exercises may be done with or without a Pilates machine. Key principles include:

- Mental focus (the all-important mind-body connection). Conscious control improves movement efficiency and muscle control.

- Central thinking. Focusing inside the mind keeps the body calm. Focusing on the torso (abdominal muscles, pelvic girdle, lower back, and "glutes") helps develop a strong core and enables the rest of the body to function efficiently.

- Alignment. Keeping the body properly aligned with a neutral spine is important for good posture.

- Stability. Before you move you have to be stable, the starting place for mobility.

- Form. Pilates is more about form than completing sets of repetitions.

- Breathing. Deep, intense breathing activates deep muscle control and keeps you focused.

- Fluidity. Graceful, nonstop motion characterizes Pilates, rather than forced repetitions.

- Integration. Several different muscle groups are engaged simultaneously to control and support movement.

Practicing Pilates regularly—and correctly—may yield a variety of benefits, including decreased pain, increased lung capacity, improved circulation, better balance and coordination, improved flexibility, and increased strength.

YOGA

Yoga is a Sanskrit word meaning "union." It can be thought of as a form of exercise developed over thousands of years in India. It promotes health and happiness by working on the mind, body, and spirit. Yogis practiced yoga exercises to join their inner spirit with the spirit of the universe. Originally, the *asanas* (postures) were developed to prepare the body so a person could sit perfectly still to meditate. Yoga is being used more frequently as a treatment modality. Where the techniques and benefits of yoga were once in doubt as a therapy, physicians are now turning to it as a viable treatment for many different conditions, including pain. Study after study has shown that for many people, yoga is one of the most effective treatments for increasing mobility and reducing pain.

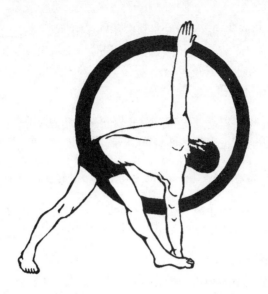

Yoga works on stretching and strengthening the body. By increasing strength, improving flexibility, and ridding the body of muscle tension, you can bring your body into balance and ease your pain. Practicing yoga can allow you to focus on positive aspects of life, as opposed to focusing strictly on pain. Deep breathing has physical and psychological benefits that can help calm the extreme emotional effects of chronic pain.

Yoga Alliance, a nonprofit organization devoted to the discipline, lists ten ways that yoga can benefit a person's health:*

1   Stress relief. By encouraging relaxation, yoga helps lower the levels of the stress hormone cortisol. Related benefits include lowering blood pressure and heart rate, improving digestion, and boosting the immune system, as well as easing symptoms of conditions such as anxiety, depression, fatigue, asthma, and insomnia.

2   Pain relief. Studies have shown that practicing *asanas*, meditation, or a combination of the two reduces pain for people with any number of conditions. Some practitioners report that emotional pain can be eased through the practice of yoga.

*Adapted from "Top 10 Reasons to Try Yoga," used with permission, yogaalliance.org. Copyright © 2006 Yoga Alliance.

3   Better breathing. Yoga teaches people to take slower, deeper breaths. This helps to improve lung function, trigger the body's relaxation response, and increase the amount of oxygen available to the body.

4   Flexibility. Improving flexibility and mobility and increasing range of movement will reduce a person's aches and pains. Yoga helps improve body alignment, resulting in better posture and helping to relieve back, neck, joint, and muscle problems.

5   Increased strength. Yoga postures use every muscle in the body, helping to increase strength. They also help relieve muscle tension.

6   Weight management. Yoga can aid in weight-control efforts by reducing cortisol levels, as well as by burning excess calories and reducing stress. Yoga encourages healthy eating habits and provides a sense of well-being and self-esteem.

7   Improved circulation. Yoga helps improve circulation and moves more oxygenated blood to the body's cells.

8   Cardiovascular conditioning. Even gentle yoga practices can provide cardiovascular benefits by lowering resting heart rate, increasing endurance, and improving oxygen uptake during exercise.

9   Focus on the present. Yoga helps practitioners to focus on the present, to become more aware, and to create better mind-body health. It improves concentration, coordination, reaction time, and memory.

10 Inner peace. The meditative aspects of yoga help many reach a deeper, more spiritual, and more satisfying place in their lives.

Throughout the centuries several distinct forms of yoga have emerged, although they all ultimately lead to the same place. There are now hundreds, if not thousands, of different "styles" of yoga, each promoting a different path to similar conclusions. Some of the better-known schools of yoga include hatha yoga, or physical and breathing exercises; raja yoga, which represents the path of transcendental knowledge; dhyana yoga, which is meditation on the absolute; Sankhya yoga, emphasizing discrimination between matter and spirit; mantra yoga, which includes the chanting of sacred prayers; and a host of others.

Some more active styles of yoga include ananda yoga, which emphasizes consciously directing the body's life force to different organs and limbs; integral yoga, which aims to integrate the various aspects of the body and mind through a combination of postures, breathing techniques, deep relaxation, and meditation, where function is given preeminence over form; shivanda yoga, which includes a series of twelve postures, breathing exercises, relaxation, and mantra chanting; hidden language hatha yoga, which seeks to promote not only physical well-being but also self-understanding by exploring the symbolism inherent in *asanas;* and somatic yoga, which is an integrated approach to the harmonious development of body and mind based on traditional yoga principles and modern psychophysiological research.

In terms of exercise to help with pain, there are two practices of yoga that are relatively slow-paced and gentle. In Vini yoga, practitioners focus on slow stretches and deep breathing. This approach often is used to treat back and arthritis pain. Iyengar yoga is another gentle style that focuses on precise body alignment. Different props, such as straps, blocks, and blankets, are used in Iyengar yoga.

As always, I recommend checking with your doctor before beginning any type of exercise program, including yoga. Additionally, it's always important to let your yoga instructor know of any problems you might have. It is a mistake to exceed your capabilities and injure yourself, though you may be able to push yourself and learn about you in the process. Just keep in mind a common saying in some twelve-step programs: "Easy does it."

ACUPUNCTURE

Practitioners of acupuncture believe illness, including chronic pain, is due to imbalances of energy in the body. Acupuncture is a component of traditional Chinese medicine in which the body is seen as a balance of two opposing and inseparable forces or energy—yin and yang. Yin

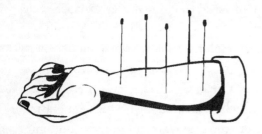

represents cold, slow, or passive aspects of the person, while yang represents hot, excited, or active aspects. Yin is masculine and yang is feminine energy. This energy is also known as **chi**, the life force that permeates the world. Health is achieved through balancing of yin and yang, and disease is caused by an imbalance of these forces, leading to a blockage in the flow of chi.

In acupuncture, hair-thin steel needles are inserted into the body to stimulate fourteen energy-carrying channels to correct the imbalances. Acupuncture is thought to relieve pain by increasing the release of endorphins, the natural chemicals in the body that block and treat pain. The acupuncturist inserts the needles into the body at predetermined points where they stay for differing lengths of time. They can be spun, warmed, or electrically energized to intensify the treatment. Some people feel energized after a treatment, while others feel relaxed.

Acupuncture is very effective at treating chronic pain including back, neck, and muscle pain, headache, facial pain, arthritis, and shingles. Acupuncturists believe treatments can strengthen the body's immune system. Acupuncture also has been used to treat obesity, drug addiction, and many other conditions.

CHI KUNG

Chi Kung is a form of exercise developed by the Chinese to enhance the mind-body connection and give you an enhanced relationship with your internal body. Also spelled Qigong, Chi Kung is the mother of Tai Chi and was developed before the martial arts influence. Practitioners of Chi Kung believe "to strain is NOT to gain," and most physical problems, including pain and diseases, are related to people being "out of balance." Chi Kung masters believe you can lessen your pain by restoring your internal/external balance.

"**Chi**" (as described in the previous section) is the powerful life-force energy and "Kung" is the power you achieve after constant practice. A master is someone who has reached mastery over his or her internal energy.

Chi Kung is moving meditation and is a very gentle form of exercise. Specific exercises help practitioners release negative energy and focus on specific areas of the body such as the spine. Chi Kung is a comprehensive program that allows students to pace themselves as they move from level to level within the discipline.

Chi Kung helps:

- Improve digestion.

- Promote relaxation and reduce stress.

- Increase flexibility and range of motion.

- Improve posture.

- Improve breathing and lung capacity.

- Enhance the cardiovascular system.

- Reduce pain.

- Lower blood pressure.

- Improve sleep.

- Increase muscle strength.

- Fight depression.

TRANSCUTANEOUS ELECTRICAL NERVE STIMULATION (TENS)

TENS units are small, battery-powered devices that produce a vibration or signal intended to interrupt pain transmissions from nerves before they reach the brain. The TENS machine can be worn outside and attached to your body via electrodes with sticky patches, or a surgeon can actually implant the electrodes under the skin. When TENS units (or electrical stimulators) are implanted, they are operated with small controls that

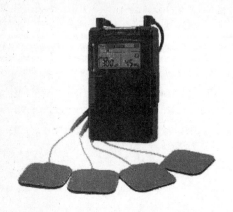

send signals through the skin into the muscles. TENS is considered to be the electrical equivalent of portable acupuncture or acupressure.

There are two theories practitioners use to explain how TENS works. The first is the gate control theory that says nerves can carry only one signal at a time, and the TENS signal overrides the pain signal, in effect closing the gate on pain transmissions before they can reach the brain. The second theory is the endorphin theory that claims TENS stimulates the body's production of these natural painkillers, giving users relief.

TENS use falls into a treatment category called "hyperstimulation analgesia." These treatments include vibration, acupressure, acupuncture, and massage. Their effectiveness as pain relievers varies among individuals, working reasonably well for some people and less so for others.

Researchers have found that the conditions most likely to get a long-term benefit from TENS include failed back syndrome, reflex sympathetic dystrophy, multiple sclerosis, peripheral vascular disease, and peripheral neuropathy.

MASSAGE

Manipulation, or massage therapy, is thousands of years old. References to massage have been found in literature from ancient China, Rome, Greece, India, and Egypt.

As a treatment, it is used in conventional medicine as well as in complementary and alternative medicine. The basic goal of the massage therapist is to increase the flow of blood and oxygen to a specific area of the body, relax and warm the soft tissues, and decrease pain by pressing, rubbing, and moving soft muscles and other tissues, primarily using the hands and fingers. The feet and forearms also are commonly used.

There are more than eighty different types of massage therapy, including:

- Swedish massage, in which the therapist uses kneading, friction, and long strokes on the muscles and joints to increase relaxation and flexibility.

- Deep-tissue massage, in which the therapist uses strokes and pressure on muscular parts of the body, focusing on the muscles deep under the skin.

- Pressure-point massage, in which the therapist applies more focused pressure on **myofascial** ("myo" refers to muscle and "fascial" refers to connective tissue) trigger points, that is, the junctions between the muscles and fascia, and uncomfortable "points" that form in the body.

People use massage for any number of reasons and health-related purposes including for general wellness, for rehabilitation, to increase relaxation, to decrease stress, to help alleviate feelings of depression or anxiety, or to relieve pain. There is no doubt that a soothing massage can ease the pain of a long day and soothe achy joints and muscles. There is growing evidence that manipulation therapy can help with chronic pain in some people. Painful conditions that have been treated with massage include cancer, back pain, fibromyalgia, neuralgia, Parkinson's disease, whiplash, and arthritis.

A variety of reasons are cited for why massage is an effective treatment for pain. Some believe that rubbing and stroking may override and block painful signals from reaching the brain—the gate control theory again. Massage clogs the pathways (closes the gate) to the brain so that pain is unable to trigger a sensation.

A number of practitioners believe that massage lessens many of the factors that contribute to the sense

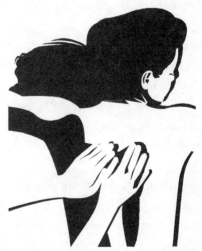

of pain, including stress, muscle tension, and spasm, and pain itself is then eased. They say that since pain and tension decrease blood circulation and massage increases it, manipulation has a negating effect on painful areas. Massage helps stimulate the limbic system to create more endorphins, the brain's natural opioid painkillers. Research with animals has shown that massage can speed the flow of **oxytocin**, a hormone that relaxes muscles and causes feelings of contentment and calmness.

Many massage techniques can be temporarily painful, as the weight of the therapist's body puts pressure on muscles, joints, and tendons to "release" them, resulting in reduction of pain. This is another example of long-term gains from short-term increase in discomfort.

AYURVEDA

Ayurveda medical practitioners believe we're all born in a state of balance. This balance is thrown out of whack by the processes of life. These disruptions can be physical, emotional, spiritual, or combinations of all these. In Ayurveda, an individual's *prakriti*, or essential "constitution," is considered to be a unique combination of physical and psychological characteristics, as well as ways in which the body's constitution functions.

Three qualities called **doshas** form important characteristics of the body and control the body's activities. The doshas are called by their original Sanskrit names: *vata*, *pitta*, and *kapha*. Each dosha is associated with a certain body type and personality type. An imbalance in any dosha may be caused by an unhealthy lifestyle or diet, too much or too little mental and physical exertion, improper digestion, or problems with how the body eliminates waste products. A person's health will be good if he or she returns to balance and has a wholesome interaction with the environment.

According to Ayurveda, a person's chances of developing certain types of diseases are related to the way doshas are balanced, the state of the physical body, and mental or lifestyle factors. Ayurveda practitioners use an individual's pulse to diagnose illness and imbalances in the body, and incorporate a variety of herbs and herbal jams to remedy an imbalanced condition. Major components of Ayurveda include a morning self-massage with warm sesame oil (*abhyanga*), meditation at sunrise and sunset, drinking small amounts of hot water throughout the day to help detoxify the body, and fasting once a week.

HYPNOTHERAPY

Hypnotherapy uses concentration, relaxation, and focused attention to attain a heightened state of awareness called a trance or hypnotic state. The person in the trance becomes able to block out outside stimuli and concentrate on specific tasks or thoughts. It is used to help people perceive stimuli differently, such as by blocking the perception of pain.

Hypnotherapy is used in two ways:

- Suggestion therapy: Being hypnotized helps a person respond to suggestions from the therapist. It can help someone change his or her behavior, for example, to stop nail biting or smoking. It is particularly useful in treating pain.

- Analysis: The therapist uses the relaxed state to find the cause of a disorder or symptom, such as a traumatic past event. Once the person reveals the trauma, his or her problems can be treated in psychotherapy.

Hypnotherapy is especially useful in treating depression, post-traumatic stress disorder, phobias, fears, anxiety, stress, sleep disorders, and grief.

Hypnotherapy addresses both physical and mental causes of pain. Therapists say that hypnotherapy helps people regulate the type, strength, and amount of pain signals that reach the brain. People can reprogram their bodies to lessen the amount of pain-inducing chemicals released. Conversely, people also can learn to regulate the amount of pain-relieving endorphins.

One hypnotherapy pain remedy is called Neuro-Linguistic Programming (NLP). NLP technique was developed to help people control stress. It is called "flash," and its goal is to reprogram the mind to use stress-creating thoughts to trigger thoughts that instill relaxation. After you've mastered the practice, therapists claim that your mind instantly and automatically exchanges, in a "flash," stress thoughts for relaxing thoughts.

Evidence from a 1995 panel shows that hypnotic interventions have been extremely successful in the management of cancer pain, temporal-mandibular disorders, tension headaches, and irritable bowel syndrome. The goal of hypnotherapy in relation to chronic pain is to produce deep relaxation to lower the fear, tension, and anxiety that usually accompany pain. In many cases of chronic pain, through the use of hypnotherapy patients were able to reduce or completely stop their use of pain medication.

HYDROTHERAPY

Hydrotherapy is using water, internally and externally, to maintain health and to treat and prevent disease. According to proponents, there is no medicine on the market that can rival the beneficial physiological effects of water. Therapeutic qualities include helping with sleep, controlling body temperature, providing derivative pain relief, and acting as an anticonvulsant. Cold water can reduce a person's pulse, kill pain, and reduce temperature in minutes. Hot water can ease joint and muscle pain and increase blood flow.

Hydrotherapy has been used to reduce acute and chronic pain for conditions like back and neck pain, arthritis, fibromyalgia, and other joint pain. Water therapy can be conducted in:

- Swimming pools, where the buoyancy supports the body and negates some of the effects of gravity. This lets pain patients perform low-impact exercises. At the same time, the water provides resistance and help in building strength and endurance.

- A "Hubbard tank" in which a person immerses his or her entire body. The water inside the tank can be raised or lowered to aid in the treatment. Convection heating can facilitate exercises to treat pain and increase blood circulation. Electrolytes can be added to the water in the Hubbard tank, which is especially beneficial for burn patients.

- Sitz baths, where the patient sits in a small tub with water covering his or her hips. These baths are used to treat lumbar pain, pelvic pain, prostatitis, and testicular pain.

- Whirlpool therapy, which uses heated, churning water that can ease aching muscles, help chronic spinal conditions, and aid in relaxation.

- Saunas and steam baths, which can relieve stress and relax muscle strains.

- Hot or cold packs that can help reduce back, facial, and limb pain.

REIKI

Reiki promotes good health through relaxation, stress relief, and pain management. In reiki, "universal life-force energy" is transmitted through the hands of a therapist from the vast pool of energy that abounds in the universe. Also called "palm healing" and "energy medicine," reiki is made up of two Japanese words: *rei*, meaning universal spirit or spiritual wisdom, and *ki*, meaning energy or life-force energy.

In CAM, energy therapies are based on the assumption that illness and pain are caused by disturbances in a person's energy. Reiki practitioners seek to improve the flow and balance of positive energy and reduce negative energy in a way that is beneficial to clients.

Although its exact origin is not known, some traditional masters teach that Dr. Mikao Usui, a Japanese physician and monk, was meditating on Mount Kurama and received his "enlightenment" for reiki. This probably occurred in the early 1900s. He started his first school for reiki in 1922. It was not used extensively in the West until the late 1930s.

Traditionally, there are three levels of reiki: reiki one, reiki two, and reiki master. Reiki is normally taught by a reiki master and involves a transfer of knowledge about how the body works and the human energy system. Becoming a reiki master can take as long as a few days to many years.

When performing reiki, the therapist poses his or her hands in twelve to fifteen different positions above the client. The hands are palms down, with the fingers and thumbs extended. Each hand position is maintained until the therapist feels the flow of energy slow or stop. Some practitioners believe they are helped by "spirit guides" that help them focus the energy flow. A treatment can last an hour or longer. There is no pressure on the body because the therapist never actually touches the client. The energy flows wherever it is needed and often is reported as a warm sensation or tingling in the body. Most report being extremely relaxed after a reiki treatment.

Practitioners report that reiki therapy:

- Promotes natural healing.

- Balances the body's energy.

- Balances the organs and glands.

- Strengthens the immune system.

- Treats symptoms and causes of illness.

- Relieves pain.

- Clears toxins from the body.

- Heals holistically.

- Releases blocked feelings.

- Promotes positive thinking.

- Helps creativity.

- Adapts to the therapy receiver.

- Enhances awareness.

- Reduces stress.

Reiki treatments have been used to reduce chronic pain, help with recovery from anesthesia and surgery, improve immunity, improve mental clarity, and lower a person's heart rate. Reiki practitioners often report clients experiencing a "cleansing crisis" after a session, in which they have feelings of nausea, tiredness, or weakness because of the release of energy toxins.

BIOFEEDBACK

Biofeedback is a technique by which people learn to control some normally involuntary processes such as muscle tension, blood pressure, and the perception of pain. Scientists believe that the relaxation effects account for a large part of the positive outcomes from using biofeedback.

There is a large amount of research literature identifying specific brain processes and physiological mechanisms that mediate the effects of biofeedback. The effectiveness of biofeedback in treating many conditions by modifying brain processes and muscle control is confirmed by this research.

In general, those who benefit most from biofeedback have conditions that are brought on or are made worse by stress such as chronic pain or high blood pressure. Biofeedback also is useful in alleviating some conditions that are not stress-related, such as attention-deficit/hyperactivity disorder (AD/HD), autism, and traumatic brain injury.

Some common forms of biofeedback therapy include:

- Electromyography (EMG), which measures muscle tension.

- Thermal biofeedback, which measures skin temperature.

- Neurofeedback or electroencephalography (EEG), which measures brain waves.

- Galvanic skin response, where sensors measure changes in skin conductivity or resistance, which is affected by the activity of a person's sweat glands and the amount of perspiration on the skin. This procedure can indicate the amount of anxiety a person is experiencing.

- Peripheral skin temperature, where a person's skin temperature is measured to assess stress level.

In a biofeedback session, electrodes from a measuring device such as the EEG or the EMG are connected to the skin of a patient. Information collected from the person is processed by the individual machine and expressed in sound or by light waves across a computer grid. A therapist then leads the person in mental exercises designed to help him or her control a particular function of his or her body, which ultimately alters the sound or light waves coming from the machine.

For example, when your muscle tension is measured by an EMG, the machine may produce a sound like a high whistle. You can learn to relate the sound to the tension in your body. By learning and performing certain exercises, you can change your muscle tension, which will lower the tone of the whistle. This relaxation technique can help lessen neck and back pain, headaches, and teeth grinding.

Biofeedback may decrease your need for medication by putting you in control of your own pain perception. The therapy seems to be very effective for some, but others have trouble mastering the necessary techniques or simply do not find relief from the procedure.

MAGNET THERAPY

Magnets have been used for centuries to treat a variety of conditions including arthritis, painful swollen joints, and blood diseases. By the third century AD, Greeks were using magnetic rings to treat arthritis and magnetic pills to stop bleeding. In the Middle Ages, magnets were used to treat poisonings and gout, and to probe and clean wounds. Doctors used magnets to pull arrowheads and other metal objects from the bodies of injured patients.

In the twentieth and twenty-first centuries, magnets are being used to treat pain, respiratory problems, high blood pressure, circulatory problems, arthritis, and stress. Scientific evidence for their effectiveness as a pain treatment is spotty at best, although there are users who swear by them. Conservative estimates say Americans spend more than $500 million a year for magnet therapy.

Most modern medical practitioners are uncommitted on magnet therapy. Even for practitioners who insist magnets relieve pain, why the magnets work is still a mystery. Some theorize that magnets may change how cells function, change how the brain processes pain, raise the temperature of the area being treated by the magnets, restore the equilibrium between cell growth and death, change how nerves transmit pain signals, and/or have an effect on the iron content in blood.

In 1979, the Food and Drug Administration approved using electromagnets to treat bone fractures that did not heal well. Some doctors use magnetic stimulation to help bone grafts heal following orthopedic surgery.

In general, practitioners place magnets with a constant flow of energy in contact with the area of the body they wish to affect. This "static magnet treatment" is being used in a number of different ways, including having the magnets in clothing, belts, jewelry, and beds.

EYE MOVEMENT DESENSITIZATION AND REPROCESSING (EMDR)

EMDR is a new method of psychotherapy developed by Dr. Francine Shapiro in the late 1980s to treat a variety of disorders. From its infancy, EMDR evolved through contributions from many different sources until it is now a full set of protocols incorporating several different therapy approaches.

No one is exactly sure how EMDR works. Research has suggested that when a person is experiencing severe trauma or chronic pain, his or her brain cannot process data in an ordinary manner. Experiences become "frozen in time," and distressing memories and feelings are relived over and over. There is no apparent improvement. These memories have a lasting negative impact on the way the person sees and relates to other people and the world in general. This can significantly interfere with that person's ability to live life.

It appears EMDR directly affects brain functions by reducing or relieving the stress associated with traumatic memories. The bilateral stimulation used in the therapy triggers brain activity normally associated with the type of information processing that occurs in REM (rapid eye movement) sleep. After successful EMDR treatment, normal information processing is resumed, as indicated in the way you experience pain. It's as though the therapy has changed the way you remember to experience pain.

In addition to being a new approach to treating chronic pain, EMDR is being used to relieve the symptoms of post-traumatic stress disorder, stress, depression, anger, existential angst, performance anxiety, and social phobias or social anxiety disorders.

Phyllis had some trepidation about undergoing EMDR when her therapist suggested it. But she simply couldn't keep living with the intense memories of her father molesting her. She was easily startled, slept poorly, and was depressed. Her pain had reemerged and seemed worse than ever, all triggered by the memories of the abuse she suffered at the hands of her father.

She found, after several sessions over a few months, that her responses to the memories subsided. They didn't disappear, as she had hoped. Truly only one thing had ever made the memories disappear, and that was to get "blotto" drunk or inject heroin or Dilaudid. But she found that after

EMDR the emotional charge of the memory was diminished. With the emotional charge lessened, Phyllis's body responded accordingly and her pain decreased again to a manageable level.

And she hadn't gotten intoxicated. She was still in recovery—after almost two and a half years.

AROMATHERAPY

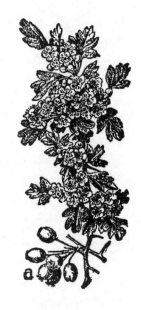

Aromatherapy literally means the therapeutic use of scents to change moods. Practitioners use essential oils distilled from plants, flowers, trees, bark, grasses, seeds, and fruits to treat a variety of ailments including fatigue, tension, stress, and, most importantly here, pain. When inhaled, aromas work on the brain and central nervous system through the olfactory (smelling) nerves. The brain's limbic system is stimulated when cells in the upper nose are exposed to odors contained in the essential aromatherapy oils. It is the same principle as when your hunger starts just as you sniff the wafting aroma of chocolate chip cookies fresh out of the oven.

Aromatherapy has been used by ancient cultures for at least 6,000 years. The ancient Romans, Egyptians, and Greeks all used aromatherapy. Hippocrates, the father of modern medicine, used aromatherapy to rid Athens of the plague. Imhotep, an ancient Egyptian healer, recommended essential oils be used in massage, baths, and embalming of the dead.

Aromatherapy is one of the oldest forms of CAM. It is also one of the fastest-growing natural remedies being used today. It works by awakening and strengthening the self-healing ability of the body. Smells can have a profound effect on your sense of well-being and body balance. Practitioners say the essential oils used in aromatherapy are antiseptic, antidepressant, antiviral, anti-inflammatory detoxifying, expectorant, and analgesic. Because essential oils are extremely concentrated, most oils require being diluted with carrier oils such as almond or grape seed oil prior to application.

There are about 150 essential oils and they can be applied directly to the skin through massage (diluted as mentioned above). A few drops of these oils also can be inhaled when placed in a bowl of warm water or in a bath, a humidifier, a diffusion device, or melted candle wax. Significant research studies have proven the therapeutic effects of aromatherapy when used to treat women after childbirth, elderly patients who suffer from insomnia, and patients who are under a great deal of stress.

Some uses of the healing properties of essential oils include lavender and lemongrass oil in the treatment of pain; chamomile, juniper, and tea tree oil to treat pain through their anti-inflammatory properties; orange, tangerine, geranium, and sage to treat high blood pressure; eucalyptus, lavender, lemon, tea tree, and basil to treat cuts and wounds; bergamot, chamomile, clary sage, rose, and sandalwood to help promote sleep; and bergamot, chamomile, rose, and valerian oil to help relieve stress.

Aromatherapy can be used to treat almost any condition that would be improved by stimulation, calming, or balancing and is often used in combination with other methods mentioned here.

OXYGEN THERAPY

More than any other element, oxygen is vital to life and good health. We can live without food or water for days, but if we don't have oxygen we will die within minutes. Every activity of our bodies, from breathing to brain function to healing to waste elimination, is regulated by oxygen.

Oxygen therapy is a number of related therapies that seek to promote healing and better health by flooding the body with oxygen. It is a holistic treatment used for detoxification and stimulation of the immune system. For many conventional physicians, it is highly controversial. Basically, practitioners believe that by controlling diseases in the body through oxygen therapy, we also can control their effects on our body's internal systems such as pain.

Proponents of oxygen therapy explain that pain starts when cells are exposed to decreased levels of oxygen, and chronic pain is driven by the absence of oxygen. It is a signal from the brain that the cell is not getting enough oxygen. This low level of oxygen in the blood is called **hypoxia**. Nerves are extremely sensitive to cellular oxygen levels. A tiny reduction can cause numbness, pain, tingling, and weakness. Therefore, the best way to optimize health is to oxygenate all your body's cells.

Naturally the best, cheapest, and most effective way to get oxygen therapy is through proper breathing. This can be cultivated and enhanced by many of the techniques already covered in this chapter.

In general, there are three therapies involving oxygen, including ozone or activated oxygen therapy, hyperbaric oxygen therapy, and hydrogen peroxide therapy. In all cases involving oxygen therapy, interested persons should first contact their doctor.

Ozone has been used in medical settings since its discovery in 1838 by Christian Friedrich Schönbein. It was used to disinfect operating rooms and surgical equipment. By the end of the nineteenth century into the first part of the twentieth century, it was used for diseases like tuberculosis and chronic middle-ear deafness. There is ongoing research on the effectiveness of ozone in other settings, but for now its use is very limited.

Hydrogen peroxide therapy has been called cutting-edge treatment by many CAM practitioners who advocate its use to treat many different illnesses including cancer, MDS, and tumors. Dr. Edward Carl Rosenow (1875–1966) developed a technique using hydrogen peroxide therapy as a way to introduce oxygen into the body to eliminate or control a host of microorganisms that he believed were the cause of many human illnesses. Introducing hydrogen peroxide into the body can be done through the use of humidifiers, baths, sprays, vegetable soaks, and as a mouthwash, to name a few.

In hyperbaric oxygen therapy (HBOT), people are exposed to high concentrations of oxygen at pressures higher than the atmosphere's in specially built chambers. In the United States, approved uses of HBOT include treatment of wounds, carbon monoxide poisoning, decompression sickness frequently suffered by underwater divers, acute crush injuries, compromised skin grafts or flaps, severe infections, and severe anemia where transfusions are not available.

MUSIC THERAPY

Music therapy is the clinical use of music to treat patients with physical, psychological, cognitive, and social functioning issues. It is a powerful and noninvasive method to reduce pain, anxiety, and depression. The treatment is for patients of all ages, with outcomes based on the individual's emotional, cognitive, and interpersonal responsiveness to the music and/or therapy relationship. The American Music Therapy Association, Inc. says the therapy has been shown to be effective for pain patients.

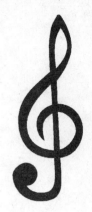

The therapy has been used for pain management, physical rehabilitation, cardiac conditions, medical and surgical procedures, obstetrics, oncology treatment, and burn debridement. As a form of sensory stimulation, music provokes responses based on familiarity, predictability, and feelings of security. Therapists use musical activities, both instrumental and vocal, to cause changes in a patient's condition. Music treatment has been used to:

- Reduce stress and anxiety.

- Help patients manage pain without drugs.

- Encourage positive changes in mood and emotional states.

- Shorten patients' stays in clinical or hospital situations.

Music helps patients deal with pain by improving respiration, lowering blood pressure, improving heart output, and easing muscle tension. According to Suzanne Hanser, Ed.D., MT-CC, of the Berklee College of Music (the world's largest independent music college located in Boston, Massachusetts), music directs a person's attention away from the pain, helps with deep rhythmic breathing, cues positive imagery, and helps patients to focus on positive thoughts and feelings.

As Phyllis, Sam, and Paul have learned, you will find a number of treatments that are effective for diminishing your pain for a time and perhaps for longer. Be diligent, open, curious, and willing.

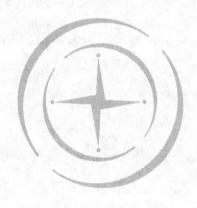

CHAPTER 11

Letting Go

Finding Harmony with Your Mind, Body, and Spirit

*"The sensual and spiritual are linked together
by a mysterious bond, sensed by our emotions,
though hidden from our eyes."*

Karl Wilhelm von Humboldt

Throughout this book I've discussed the various components of chronic pain and suffering and examined how they can affect your mind and body. I have also provided a number of methods and exercises that have the potential to alleviate some of the ongoing symptoms associated with chronic pain. One of the goals of this book is to help you learn how to live with chronic pain by looking at all aspects comprising your psychological and physical makeup. In this chapter, I'll explore how a different force in your life—your spirit—can play a role in helping you find freedom from the daily chaos of living in chronic pain.

The concept of spirituality is often looked at as synonymous with religion. Nothing could be further from the truth. Many spiritual leaders of today and from the past, as well as individuals who are on a spiritual quest, have no affiliation whatsoever with a religion. They simply embrace a gentle and benevolent manner of living in a world rife with hatred, bigotry, and man's inhumanity to man. To differentiate between these two concepts, it might be helpful if I first gave some broad definitions of religion and spirituality.

Religion generally means a constructed set of fundamental beliefs and rituals that offer veneration to and reverence for a supernatural power(s) or entity that controls human destiny. Most religions contain moral codes governing human affairs. The belief in a supreme being is as old as humankind, and as a result there are thousands of different religions in existence today, with a thousand more offshoots. Common examples of religions are Christianity with its Ten Commandments and holy book, the Bible; Judaism and the Torah; Islam and the Quran, or Koran; and Hinduism, which is considered the oldest religion in the world and has four sacred texts called Vedas, meaning knowledge.

Many religious teachings acknowledge that all spiritual principles are alike or even the same. After all, think about the "right" way to live. Buddhism calls this right speech, right actions, and right livelihood. Toltec wisdom calls it the four agreements: Be impeccable with your word; don't take anything personally; don't make assumptions; and always do your best. Christianity says "love thy neighbor as thyself" and "turn the other cheek." Judaism teaches "that which is hateful to yourself, do not do to others." Those who practice Taoism believe one should "love the world as your own self; then you can truly care for all things." Many people do find spirituality in their religion, and if this is so for you, I encourage you to actively participate in religious activities.

Spirituality can be thought of as "religion without the rules."

Can you see the similarities? Spirituality can be thought of as "religion without the rules." It is the ways you want to live and pertains to the intellectual or higher endowments of the mind or soul. It is not tangible or of the material world. In seeking spirituality, one looks inward to reflect on his or her place in the universe, seeing that each individual is part of the greater whole. It can be said that spirituality is reaching for the consciousness of your humanness and accepting that you truly are an extension of the universe. It seems to be a lofty goal to reach for, but as you become more aware and mindful of yourself and your humanity, you begin to feel a sense of peace and harmony with yourself, the world around you, and those who populate it.

What this has to do with pain relief is that living a contented life without heaps of guilt and shame, with a sense of meaning and purpose, and with an eye for others as well as yourself, is the road to less suffering.

Take some time right now to list some spiritual values that make sense to you and would be helpful to you along your journey.

If you refer back to some of the research presented in earlier chapters about the brain and how it affects the body, you will see how being bunched and knotted up with pain, physically and mentally, can cause you to feel pain more intensely. It's how the nervous system is wired. Between releasing chemicals that create feelings and becoming used to maladaptive behaviors, your body takes the brunt of these reactions and the pain not only intensifies, but persists for longer periods.

Being in relentless and agonizing pain takes a toll on your body. It stresses the body and can cause myriad health concerns and problems. It often leads to distress. For instance, stress causes a chemical reaction within the brain's cortex and limbic system. Continued and excessive stress, like that experienced with chronic pain, causes pathological changes of the cortex and limbic system, resulting in a number of conditions that ultimately diminish mental and physical functioning.

Continued stress can lead to headache, upset stomach, high blood pressure, and sleeping problems, to name a few. It's an unwanted and terrible addition to the troubles you already have with chronic pain. Stress is the final boulder that, when added to your already mounting tower of symptoms and associated chronic pain conditions, can cause life to tumble down and crush you. Pain has engulfed your life, and the search for relief has created a cycle of chaos. There seems to be no way out; you feel trapped.

Seeking Balance and Harmony

This is where seeking balance and harmony through spiritual practices comes in. I am suggesting that you let go of your pain on a deeper level. This is not easy, and it can be difficult to comprehend. It takes courage and faith to trust in the process of releasing your attachment to your pain. In turn, you will find that your pain releases its hold on you. I challenge you to give up what is not helping you—your pain.

The Chronic Pain Recovery Program at Las Vegas Recovery Center is based on abstinence from opioids. As medical director, I've seen many successful examples of people who stop their medications under medical supervision and improve dramatically. One of the first steps in this program is to recognize that your pain is no longer just physical, but also emotional and spiritual. You need to reconnect with your emotions, your body, and your spirit. You will benefit by allowing yourself to be open to the possibility of real, lasting relief without medication. Living with pain in this way is a process, and it takes time. Remember, your chronic pain did not happen overnight. It is something that developed over years. With that in mind, you will recognize that relief does not magically appear.

Life is not static. It is in flux and in motion and constantly changing with each millisecond; however, living in chronic pain can make life seem to be an incessant repetition of agony, hopelessness, and frustration—a stagnant pool with no way out. Your journey in life, of enjoying rich and pleasurable experiences, doesn't have to stop because of chronic pain. You can create a life filled with vitality and function. It won't be easy, but it can be achieved.

You may find the thought of letting go of your pain scary or even ridiculous. After all, you are not "holding on to" your pain. How can anyone think you actually want to hold on to such a negative force in your life? The pain you feel is the result of the failure of your last surgery or your joints grating against each other or your intestines burning with each swallow, not because you are holding on to it. But your pain has now become part of you. It defines you. It has consumed your identity. In other words, your pain is you; you have become your pain. This is what you must seek to let go of. The pain you feel is *not* you; it is simply the pain you feel.

Take a moment to challenge those irrational thoughts trying to convince you that you are hopeless, that no one understands, and that your pain will never go away. You are not alone, and there is hope. Though your pain will likely not be gone for good, you can experience freedom from pain a good part of the time and have less suffering in your life. Of this I can assure you.

Sam was truly "sick and tired of being sick and tired" but didn't know how to change things. His trainer had a spiritual practice based in yoga and meditation that really appealed to Sam. Actually, Sam was attracted to his trainer's mellow nature and attitude that "everything is going to be okay, because that is what will be" and an overall positive outlook on life and the world. He went to meditation group with Joe, his trainer, and met some people there who seemed to be content with their lives. Sam still struggled with accepting his lot in life with his deformed body, but with daily meditation practice, he found that he was a little softer toward himself and others. Eventually, he was able to make peace with his dad who had always been tough on Sam. They were so much alike and neither gave the other a break, until one day Sam came to a place where he could forgive. Just like that, the burden of guilt, shame, anger, and resentment seemed to evaporate. Of course, this had been coming over months of practice, but for Sam and Frank, it came as a welcome change in their relationship.

Sam didn't stop there. He went on a spiritual retreat, and started listening to tapes and reading voraciously. The more he worked at it, the more spontaneous and comfortable he became. He had a sense of peace and serenity that had eluded him for most of his life. For the first time in decades he slept well at night without sleeping pills, and his free-floating anxiety was, for the most part, gone.

Staying in the Moment

Here are a few suggestions that may help you learn to start letting go of your pain and become more mindful of your mind, body, and spirit.

- Take an active role in learning to live with your pain. Try to isolate the pain in your mind and focus on its origin. Create an object in your mind to diminish the pain. If your back pain burns with each breath you take, visualize placing ice on that part of your back. If your joints are sore, send healing breath to them. If your stomach is cramping, picture the cramps becoming looser, like a taut rubber band unwinding. There are many images you can use. Be creative!

- Focus on all that you are able to do, rather then dwelling on the things that you can no longer do. Make a gratitude list of all the good things in your life.

- Let go of your sense of being "different" and any fear you may have of other people criticizing you. Finding a support group can help diffuse your sense of being unique. After all, there are millions of people with conditions just like yours and worse.

- Do what you need to do to ease your pain (for example, taking a pillow into the movie theater with you) without worrying about what other people might think. Stand and walk around when sitting becomes uncomfortable.

- Seek and accept support from family, friends, therapists, and support groups. You don't have to do this alone.

- Extend yourself to others on the days when you feel well enough. Often getting "out of yourself" diminishes your suffering. The more you learn, the more able you will be to help someone else who is in pain with encouragement and information about your experience.

- Prioritize your life. Decide what's important and what you want to do about it, and then do it.

Another aspect of seeking spirituality or oneness with self involves meditation and/or prayer. Many books have been written on the topic of meditation and how to practice it. Choose one that appeals to you and can help you learn how to meditate. Don't get bogged down with the religious implications. Start with small steps.

Maybe you cannot sit with your legs crossed in lotus position because it makes your back hurt. Instead, find a comfortable place to sit where your back is supported, or lie down (but try not to fall asleep) and go from there. The practice here is to learn how to still your mind and try to reconnect with your spirit. You can do this anywhere, really. It's not about looking like a yogi, but rather finding a place inside you where you can make peace with your pain. Chanting, singing, and prayer may help as well, since they often tend to take the focus away from your pain and bring you to a serene place.

> *Some people living in chronic pain find*
> *that the pain is lessened when they share*
> *with other individuals who have*
> *the same experiences that they do.*

Some people living in chronic pain find that the pain is lessened when they share with other individuals who have the same experiences that they do. Many hospitals and pain management treatment centers have support groups where people in chronic pain can come to share in a common and supportive environment. This particular format is part of what makes twelve-step programs so successful. There is a unique and therapeutic quality to sharing with another person who is familiar with and understands what you've been through. An example of this is the Pain in Recovery Support Group started as a component of Las Vegas Recovery Center's Chronic Pain Recovery Program.

The Pain in Recovery Support Group is a secondary, abstinence-based support group for people who suffer and live with chronic pain. The group is not a twelve-step fellowship, but members do attend a variety of twelve-step fellowships for their primary recovery journey. The primary goal of the group is to provide a safe and nurturing environment so members can share freely without fear of judgment and learn to heal while staying on the road of recovery. Participants in the Pain in Recovery Support Group share their experiences about how they confront and manage their pain and help others to do the same.

Another concept found in twelve-step programs is powerlessness. Once members in the program admit their powerlessness over alcohol/other drugs or food or sex or gambling or whatever obsession they are engaged in, they are free to begin the recovery process. This type of admission opens the door for surrender and acceptance. This same principle can work for addressing your chronic pain. You are powerless over your pain and the circumstances that created it; however, you are not helpless. Start by telling yourself, "For this moment I will accept my circumstances relating to pain, and I will seek to turn negatives into positives. I will stop fighting against my pain today." There are solutions that can help you get back to some normalcy; you will need to find what works best for you. Remember, when resistance is decreased, pain decreases.

Phyllis rediscovered her spirituality as her pain became more manageable. She found that by giving up the fight against her fibromyalgia and back pain, as well as her addiction, she could more easily embrace life. Daily meditation, sometimes for only ten minutes, settled her down and allowed her to cope with stress, anxiety, and anger more effectively. She went to church for the first time in years and found the cadence of the prayers extremely satisfying. The payoffs were evident to her and those around her.

She was busy with twelve-step recovery and her series of activities, but the relief and joy she experienced made all the work well worth it. Phyllis felt congruent with her body, with her soul, with her God, and with the universe. She was content for the first time in a long time.

Paul struggled with spirituality. He felt abandoned by God, and religion had never served him. Rather, it got him in touch with the anger he felt toward organized religion and the guilt he felt for most of his life for being a "bad Jew." He struggled with the concept of "turning it over" to a power greater than himself that he had heard about at the twelve-step meetings he attended. In fact, before his accident he was self-sufficient and an accomplished attorney. He thought, "Who needs God or rules or more guilt?"

Then, as Paul tells it, "the strangest, most unexpected thing happened." It was a Sunday night, the house was quiet, and Paul was awakened by a jolt of excruciating pain in his back and hip. The pain didn't respond to the stretching he had learned to help relieve the spasms, but instead kept escalating. The more pain, the more panic he felt, until his heart was pounding out of his chest at 120 beats per minute (up from his usual 80). He was sweating like he had when he withdrew from the opioids a few months prior. He wanted something to take the pain away. He seriously considered waking Lila or calling 911, but instead he started to write a letter to God (a suggestion from his twelve-step sponsor just that morning).

He wrote, "Why me, God? What did I do to deserve this? I don't want to keep living this way! I'd rather die!" Paul's body was taut as, for the first time, he seriously considered ending his life. The idea that the pain would end was balanced by the fear that his body might die but the pain might carry on in his soul.

Out of some corner of his mind came a cry he had never heard before from himself: "Please help me!" He started to sob uncontrollably. He lost track of time, not sure of anything except his desperate desire for relief and help. A little later, he felt Lila's soft hand on his head, stroking his brow, silently rubbing his shoulders as he continued to cry. He looked up, finally, and saw such love in her eyes, and in that moment, he felt a weight lifted from him. His back relaxed and the pain was gone for the first time since his accident. He literally felt no pain in that moment.

To this day, Paul, who prior to that night had considered himself an agnostic, still is baffled by what happened. He did know that he had over an hour of total relief from his pain. Though it returned in the days to come, it was not as severe, and his response to it was different. He felt calmer and more accepting. Lila and her family said Paul seemed like he'd gone through something and come out the other side. His sponsor, who is religious and a strong believer in God, told Paul he'd had a "spiritual experience."

Paul wasn't sure, and didn't much care what the explanation was for the shift in his consciousness about his pain. He liked the change and began working earnestly on practicing techniques that would help him on his process of pain recovery.

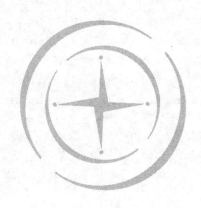

CHAPTER 12

Time Takes Time

"Happiness, not in another place but this place . . .
not for another hour, but this hour."

Walt Whitman

Time means different things to different people at different moments. Think about your experience with time as you waited for a desired event—a graduation, wedding, or party. The time creeps up slowly and you feel like the day will never arrive. Then it's over in a flash; all that's left is a memory. As a youngster, each year is a huge increment of your life; as a senior, each year is a mere fraction. Life has passed, and your memories are a flashing slide show.

Time occurs a moment, a breath, a minute at a time. Endless waiting, and then over before you know it. Hours pass so slowly, they seem never-ending. It's relative, of course. Einstein said time and space are part of a continuum.

Pain is a similar story. If your pain is here, in this moment, you can be okay with it by taking a breath, stretching, distracting yourself, and getting on with your day. If you get caught up in the "endless nature of my chronic pain, which will be with me till I die," as Paul, Sam, and Phyllis had done in the past, then each moment becomes frustrating and hopeless with unrelenting pain.

The difference is in your attitude. Even there, you will find a different perception of time on a different day. It's the nature of your reality. As with everything you've learned in this book so far, a little effort at a time will go a long way. Pacing yourself, taking small steps, and being gentle with yourself as you move through your day, you'll come to realize that a breath at a time is the key to finding the calm and peace of pain-free moments. Practicing and developing patterns of behavior will take time as well, and eventually new patterns will be established. Persistence over time will result in changes in your experience of pain.

If you've taken the time to read *A Day without Pain*, you may be able to understand that time is not necessarily an unavoidable march toward more pain. Today, you may be able to accept that you can actually change how you feel, that if you give yourself time you can alter your experience of pain and lessen its impact on your body and in your life.

This book was written to help you help yourself.

This book was written to help you help yourself. In it I have attempted to describe what pain is: acute and chronic. I explained that your brain is plastic in that it is changeable, adaptable. I have illustrated how pain can and probably has changed your brain and the way it works. I have described how your emotions are intertwined with pain like two sides of the same coin. Your emotions have a huge impact on your experience of pain. I have suggested that since pain changed your brain, it is possible for you to consciously make further changes, to alter your brain and thereby alter your experience of pain.

I described why medications are very often the favorite method of treatment for pain, and I examined some of the problems associated with them, including addiction. Then I revealed how chronic pain is not a one-person problem. Pain is something that has a major impact on the entire family. I described how families can be affected when one member is afflicted with pain.

I offered a detailed list of more than two dozen different alternative methods for treating pain. I described how these methods work and the painful conditions that have been successfully treated by them. The methods described here can help reduce your pain, if you give them time to work. Finally, I offered suggestions for how you can incorporate spirituality into your journey toward reduction of pain.

Once Sam decided to come off the medications, he had to put up with a lot—new sensations of aching in the morning, stiffness as he began the stretches that he had learned, and occasionally a shooting sensation into his right foot that made him think he was being shocked with 10,000 volts of electricity (he liked to exaggerate).

The withdrawal from the medications felt endless, but looking back, it lasted only a few weeks. He was fascinated by how his mind responded while he was in the midst of the detoxification process, and now, four months later, the way his mind was able to note it as a distant memory. It reinforced that he never wanted to go through that again, but his suffering from the withdrawals was over.

To make matters better, he noticed things in his new drug-free state that were exhilarating. The blue of the sky, the sound of the birds, the touch of a friend's hand, the sound of his favorite music—all of these were perceived by his senses in a way that he hadn't experienced for years. When he became frustrated with the slight weakness in his right leg, he balanced it by knowing that with every passing week, he grew stronger, lifting heavier weights at the gym. And with the increasing strength, he noticed that ever so slowly the pain lessened, the stiffness was a bit less bothersome, and the electric shocks were now only 2,000 volts.

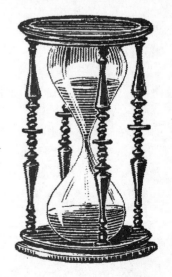

He was amazed that as time passed his life got better, both physically and emotionally. As he made room for the pain in his life, he found that he suffered less. He would find himself thinking how much better his life would have been if only he had known this years ago. Then he would find himself drawn to regret. But he would gently ease himself back to the present and feel excitement for the potential that lay ahead. Over the past six months he had accomplished so much. He gave up all the drugs, exercised to the point of excelling in yoga, took power walks daily, and was thinking of doing a half-marathon. His life had changed dramatically in such a relatively short time, and he could only imagine how much better it could be. "Truly, all I have is today, this moment, this breath," Sam repeated as he settled in to meditate before his daily run.

Paul's recovery was too slow for him and Lila. Now that he had seen what he was capable of, he wanted it all back, *now*. An injury while he was playing basketball brought them both up short. They met with their therapist who helped them see that their impatience was natural, but it had to be subdued lest they fail to move beyond where they were. Their relationship with each other was like they were meeting for the first time. Lila had grown during the years of Paul's disability and addiction, and now that he was back in her life as a fully functional human being, she would have to make room for him. She wanted the "old Paul" back, she'd say, but actually, as their therapist pointed out, that's not really what she wanted.

The "new Paul" was a bit more tentative and less self-assured. He had been through hell and was back with the living. Getting to know each other was taking longer than she had imagined and was much tougher in some ways than it was when he was "gone." She had to interact directly with him now after she had grown used to relying only on herself. Over the months in couples therapy, they learned to negotiate with each other, sorting through the maze of recovery.

She didn't want to go back to the way it was, but she was unsure of where and how they fit together anymore. Gradually, as Lila and Paul learned to be patient with each other, they developed a new relationship, better and different than anything they had experienced previously. To the great satisfaction of both of them, they were able to be more effective parents to their son. Paul was able to pass along a powerful message to others who suffered from chronic pain and were struggling with drug abuse. He attended twelve-step support meetings, and over time developed a reputation for being a role model for those with pain and addiction. Lila and Paul were living in recovery, a day at a time.

Although chronic pain can appear in the blink of an eye, in most cases it takes time for it to fully develop. Phyllis's pain didn't explode into her life full-blown, but appeared slowly, over time, until she was overwhelmed. It took time for it to build up. She learned about pain early from her bedridden mother and her abusive father. She developed several painful conditions of her own—fibromyalgia and arthritis—as she grew into young adulthood. Addiction to drugs complicated her life immeasurably, and through recovery she found her own way back to herself. Phyllis worked hard to reframe her experience of pain, and grew to realize that her physical pain was inextricably linked with her emotional pain. Her relief came through self-knowledge, restoring of her faith, meditative practices, and hard work; it was time-consuming, but it had great payoffs.

As Fast as Possible

Time is not a cure for chronic pain, but it can be crucial for improvement. It takes time to change, to recover, and to make progress. While it's unlikely (though not impossible) that the treatment methods outlined in this book would immediately result in pain reduction, if you give them time to work, you might be pleasantly surprised. It's progress if every day for three years you rate your pain as a six on a scale of one to ten, and one day after meditation you drop it to a five. It took time, but you improved. It's progress if you normally spend twelve hours in bed all day, every day, and one day after a month of stretching and soothing baths you find you are up and about more than reclining.

It takes time to change, to recover,
and to make progress.

Exercise is one of the most effective treatment methods available to those in chronic pain. Whether Pilates, Chi Kung, yoga, or any other form of regulated movement, exercise has been proven to help ease pain by lengthening and strengthening muscles, relaxing tension, and increasing flexibility. But it takes time to work.

Insomnia is an extremely common problem for those who have chronic pain. Studies have proven that merely changing the aroma inhaled every night can help with sleep and therefore help reduce pain. But it takes more than just one night to work. It may take weeks or months; it takes time.

Chronic pain can rob you of yesterday, today, and tomorrow; it robs you of time. Nothing can give you back the moments lost to the experience of pain, but it is my belief that the suggestions in *A Day without Pain* can give you hope for a future in which time becomes hope—hope for a pain-free tomorrow.

So there you have it—time takes time. No easy fix for this problem, that's for sure. Some of you tried to find such a solution in medication and found that this plan backfired. You could get some short-term relief from medications, but nothing that lasted and not without a price. The alternative is to first believe there is another way to live. There is, I assure you. Anyone with chronic pain can live more fully as he or she learns to cultivate mindfulness, stress reduction, acceptance, and positive regard. These skills are developed like muscles and will eventually replace the old, worn-out beliefs of "poor me," "it's never going to get better," and "I can't do it" that many of you live with in the chronic pain syndrome. Practice these diligently and your life *will* change.

You will notice a decrease in your pain, and certainly you will suffer less. This change is in your hands and in your control if you choose to exercise it. Physical modalities for chronic pain abound, and I encourage you to pick a few and work them with your body. Find some you feel are helpful. Be gentle with yourself. Don't be a taskmaster or a judge or a jury. Get on your own side. The pain, it turns out, is a product of your limbic system—a construct of your defense system against the pain, which has turned against you. As you realize this, you will see the pain inside you dissolve, like ice to water to vapor.

I wish you many days without pain.

Las Vegas Recovery Center Chronic Pain Recovery Program

Outcomes and Commentary

In April 2006, the Las Vegas Recovery Center (LVRC) started accepting clients into the Chronic Pain Recovery Program (CPRP), an opioid-free program for treatment of chronic pain and symptoms of substance dependence. LVRC designed CPRP to help clients cope with and manage their chronic pain while discontinuing the use of habit-forming medications.

The recommended course of treatment for individuals who are experiencing both chronic pain and substance dependence includes seven to twenty-one days of inpatient medically managed withdrawal from opioids (Chapter Four) and any other mood-altering medications, followed by four weeks of specialized inpatient treatment for chronic pain and substance dependence. Any acute and post-acute withdrawal symptoms are treated by medical management at the center.

Once the detoxification process has been successfully completed, clients are transferred to CPRP. Clients participate in client-specific activities, all individual and group treatment activities of the inpatient rehabilitation program for substance abuse/dependence, as well as chronic pain groups. Complementary and alternative medicine (CAM) treatments and nonmood-altering, nonopioid medications are continued as indicated throughout their stay. CAM interventions are tailored for each client and are selected to target and improve chronic pain, range of motion (ROM), muscular tension, anxiety and **dysphoria**, substance abuse/dependence, substance craving, and self-directed comfort and control. During the second week, a physical therapy (PT) evaluation is performed with ongoing PT treatments for core strengthening, pain reduction, and increased activity level based on an individualized treatment plan.

The following table outlines the CAM interventions used.

Table A

Complementary and Alternative Medicine Interventions Used			
Disease or Symptom Targeted	Intervention, Frequency/ Duration	Known/Theorized Mechanism of Action	Intended Effect
Chronic Pain	1. Chiropractic, three times per week 2. Acupuncture, weekly 3. Electric stimulation, dose variable, chiropractic	1. Improved spinal alignment results in decreased pain and increased function 2. Release of endorphins and regulation of neurotransmitter balance (Tufts, EBCAM) 3. High voltage: Endorphin or enkephalin release. Microcurrent: protein synthesis. Biphasic or Russian: muscle fatigue	Decreased pain, relaxation, increased mobility
Decreased Range of Motion (ROM)/ deconditioning	1. Stretches, daily 2. Chi Kung, weekly 3. Physical Therapy (PT) 4. Yoga, daily	1. Gentle increase in ROM 2 & 3. Oxygenation of tissue, increased GABA levels 4. More rigorous weight training and core strengthening	Increased mobility and strength, relaxation, mood enhancement (endorphins), decreased pain
Muscular Tension	Massage, certified massage therapist, weekly	Improve circulation; enhance relaxation; decrease symptoms of anxiety, depression, and pain; stimulate feeling of well-being	Relaxation, muscular tension/ decreased adhesions

continued on page 183

Complementary and Alternative Medicine Interventions Used (Continued)			
Disease or Symptom Targeted	**Intervention, Frequency-Duration**	**Known/Theorized Mechanism of Action**	**Intended Effect**
Anxiety, dysphoria	Reiki, reiki master weekly	Balancing of subtle energy fields; possible electromagnetic correlations have been detected using experimental measurement devices (Tufts, 2007; EBCAM)	Relaxation, mood enhancement (endorphins)
Substance abuse/dependence	Hypnosis, clinical psychologist as ordered	General relaxation in an alpha state renders the mind less distractible and more receptive to therapeutic suggestions (Tufts, 2007; EBCAM)	Decrease pain, anxiety, and enhance therapeutic benefit of other interventions
Substance Craving	Ear laser, daily and as needed	Stimulates CNS via cranial and spinal nerves. This results in neurotransmitter release in the periaqueductal gray matter and pituitary, which modulates pain.	Decrease or eliminate craving
Self-directed Comfort and Control	1. Heat 2. Ice/cold 3. Interferential/TENS 4. Aqua jet massage bed	1. Vasodilatation to decrease pain sensation and increase metabolic rate of affected area 2. Vasoconstriction to decrease pain sensation and local edema 3 & 4. Muscle relaxation and decreased pain sensation, as well as healing through muscle stimulation and increased metabolic rate at area of treatment	Decrease pain, muscle relaxation

Chronic pain therapies include multidisciplinary educational and process groups conducted by physicians, nurses, counselors, and psychologists. Clients study from and complete assignments in a chronic pain workbook, *Pain Recovery: How to Find Balance and Reduce*

Suffering from Chronic Pain (Central Recovery Press), which focuses on the difference between physical and emotional pain, as I discussed here in Chapter Six. The workbook also teaches management and coping strategies to improve quality of life, recovery, and relapse prevention. In addition to group meetings, general interventions are used on a daily basis to help clients progress. The milieu is judged to be one of the most important factors in client improvement—seeing one client who is two weeks further in treatment is a powerful motivator and model for improvement. Working with others also underscores the human and spiritual connections that foster recovery. General interventions are discussed in Table A2.

Table A2

General Interventions Used		
Intervention	**Frequency**	**Intended Effect**
Client self-efficacy	Daily/constant	Include client as an equal team member in the management of his or her chronic pain
Cognitive behavioral therapy (CBT)/ motivational interviewing	Daily/constant (group and individual)	Assist client in reframing and learning new coping methods to deal with and minimize pain experience Assess, diagnose, and address any mental illness or somatic factors that contribute to chronic pain
Education	Daily/constant (formal and informal)	Increase client understanding of pain processes and modalities that work to relieve or reduce pain, how these modalities work, and when to use them
Peer support	Daily/constant (formal and informal)	Decrease sense of isolation/ alienation. Increase sense of community and engagement

continued on page 185

General Interventions Used (Continued)		
Intervention	**Frequency**	**Intended Effect**
Screening and psychotherapy	At admission and as needed	Systematically identify individual co-occurring PTSD, bipolar disorder, and depression in clients since initiating treatment, as these co-occurring illnesses can influence clinical outcome
Family program	Four-day intensive program	Family educated and supported to assist the client upon return home
Group meetings	Weekly	Review specific workbook assignments
Body scan/ meditation	Daily	Bring relaxed attention to various parts of the body

Client progress is tracked and measured throughout the course of the CPRP using the Pain Outcomes Profile (POP). The POP is a twenty-three-item questionnaire that utilizes eleven-point (zero to ten) numerical rating scales to assess a number of relevant dimensions in the pain patient's experience. It was developed by the American Academy of Pain Management to assess three domains of a patient's pain experience. These domains are assessed using two pain intensity scales, three self-reports of functional impairment scales, and two scales that address self-reported emotional functioning (seven scales total). The POP also contains two numerical rating scales to assess the patient's experience of pain intensity *right now* and *pain on the average during the last week*.

There are three scales in the domain of perceived functional impairment due to pain: Mobility, Activities of Daily Living (ADL), and Vitality. The Mobility scale contains four items that rate a patient's perception of pain-related interference with the ability to walk, to carry or handle everyday objects, or to climb stairs, and whether pain requires the use of assistive devices (for instance, a walking aid or wheelchair). ADLs are assessed with four items that inquire about pain-related interference with the ability to bathe, dress, use the bathroom, and manage personal grooming. The patient's subjective feeling of a lack of vitality is assessed with three items rating the ability to perform physical activities, feelings of overall energy, and strength and endurance.

Self-reported emotional functioning is assessed with two scales: Negative Affect and Fear. The Negative Affect scale contains five items, asking the patient to rate the degree to which pain affects self-esteem, feelings of depression, feelings of anxiety, ability to concentrate, and feelings of subjective tension. The Fear scale contains two items that rate how much worry is experienced about re-injury due to increasing activity and feelings of safety exercising. (American Academy of Pain Management website: www.aapainmanage.org)

Each client completes the POP upon admission to LVRC, once while in detoxification, every Wednesday thereafter, and once before discharge from the facility. For the purposes of program evaluation data from Admission, the POP closest to the middlemost date of the client's stay (Mid), and Discharge were compared by using a paired t-test statistical analysis. Results showed statistically significant improvement on all scales at both the Mid and Discharge intervals. The following figures show the average scores for each scale of the POP:

Figure A1

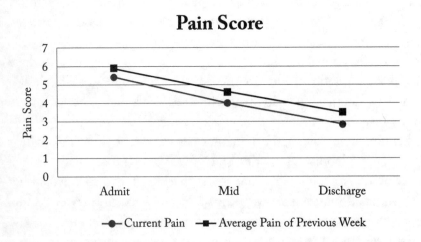

Figure A2

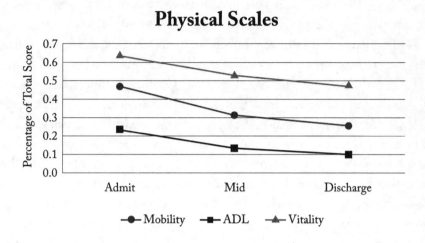

Physical Scales

Figure A3

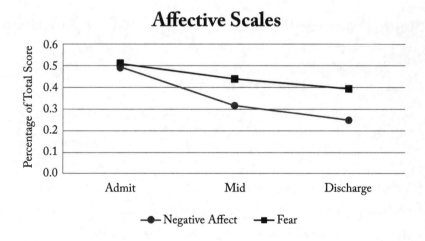

Affective Scales

The average length of stay (LOS) for clients used in the data for the previous graphs was thirty-seven days (excluding days of inpatient drug abuse rehabilitation for clients who entered the rehab program after discharging from CPRP). The average LOS in detoxification was five and one-half days, and was thirty-one days in CPRP. The average LOS for CPRP is greater than the planned twenty-eight days because clients who left the program with fewer than twenty days of treatment, including detoxification, were not included in the data. Also, there were ten clients who opted to stay longer. The maximum time spent in the CPRP program was eighty-three days. Of the thirteen clients who chose to transfer to the inpatient rehabilitation program after leaving CPRP, the average length of stay in the rehab setting was 28.54 days. The average stay of clients was forty-five days and the minimum stay was twenty-two days. In order to be included in the current sample, the recorded POP data must cover at least 75 percent of stay. Seven clients who left the program early were included in the data; all other clients were discharged from the program as planned.

Before entering the Chronic Pain Recovery Program, clients commonly report increased levels of pain despite the various treatments and surgeries they had received for their pain.

Client Testimonials

ROBERT

Q: What was your experience at LVRC like?

"The program for me was a totally different way of treating my pain than what my previous doctors or Western medicine first offered me. It was totally different."

Q: What's different for you now?

"Everything! My body is healed, and I don't have any pain. I have zero pain. I don't know if those results are common, but for me they're a reality."

Q: What would you tell others about your experience?

"Living under any kind of narcotic medication for pain is no way to live, and there are alternatives that work and work well. The staff at LVRC is sympathetic and knowledgeable of those ways. They're extremely helpful in sharing those ways to live the way I live today, which is pain-free and without narcotics. It's having a clear mind and living the right way again—living purposefully."

Q: What changes have you noticed in your life?

"I can do anything, anything. All activities are available again. I even weight-train.

Other comments:

"I didn't really understand narcotic medication and the dependency it creates."

BEN

Q: What changes have you noticed in your life?

"I've been able to live with my pain a lot better and not focus on it so much as a villain, but accept it into my life as a part of me and then set it aside and just live with it. By my accepting it in its entirety and not denying it, it doesn't slow me down as much, and I'm able to function better."

Q: Has your quality of life improved?

"My quality of life is a lot better. The pain is also less since I stopped taking narcotics."

Q: Has your level of functioning changed?

"My functioning is the same, but my pain is easier to deal with."

Q: What would you tell others about your experience?

"If you can afford it, it will help you deal with your pain. It seemed to help everyone who was in the pain program while I was there. It was definitely worth it to me."

DELORES

Q: What was your experience at LVRC like?

"I was enlightened about my relationship with pain, as well as informed about hyperalgesia. Learning about hyperalgesia was really useful because that was information I wasn't privy to before. And the fact that the drugs I was taking to help with my pain might actually be making it worse was totally new to me. It's counterintuitive, for one thing. And when you're severely addicted to a pain drug and in pain, it's the last thing you're willing to believe.

"The pain program was useful to me when I could become completely open-minded to let the information in. The information is invaluable, but until I was willing to hear the information it wasn't of much use."

Q: What's the biggest change you've noticed in your life?

"The biggest change has been that I have been able to get my physical health back."

Q: How has your quality of life changed?

"Before LVRC I didn't really have a quality of life. In an unconscious way, I felt like I was waiting to die when I got to LVRC, and now I've got a life again. I have interest in life again. I'm just in recovery for ten months, so I'm still building a lot of stuff back like my relationships, interest in work, interest in exercise, and other things. I now have a chance to have those things again. Before I got to LVRC those things that were so precious to me were falling away in my life."

Q: What would you tell others about LVRC's pain program?

"It taught me to how to have a different relationship with my pain."

Other comments:

"It's amazing how much of what was happening to me by the time I got to LVRC was really just about dependence and misguided thinking. I thought I needed the drugs to feel better, but it was all just an illusion."

RALPH

"LVRC is top-notch. The clients were great, and I couldn't have asked for a better staff. From Dr. Pohl to the nursing staff to the counselors, I would not recommend anywhere else other than LVRC.

"I've been to several different rehab centers. Most of those had doctors or staff who had never been through an addiction process. What I found at LVRC were people who had walked in my shoes, and they understood where I was coming from.

"The people at LVRC, or at least 90 percent of them, are in recovery. When you run into someone who isn't in recovery, it makes it very hard to communicate. The people at LVRC were the right kind of people.

"The massage therapy, reiki, meditation, acupuncture, and everything that I went through there really helped. At first my pain level was an eight or nine, but when I left it was maybe a three or four. It made a huge difference."

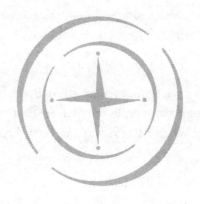

A

Ablation Removal of abnormal growths or damaging substances from the body (especially organs) by mechanical means such as surgery or the application of chemicals.

Acetylcholine The first neurotransmitter ever identified. It is involved with voluntary movement by stimulating muscle contraction and exciting nerves.

Active release Soft-tissue treatment for problems that occur with muscles, tendons, ligaments, and nerves.

Adjuvants Medications that have a primary use other than pain relief, but are often helpful in easing pain. They include antidepressants, muscle relaxants, and anticonvulsants.

Advil Brand name for generic drug ibuprofen, a nonsteroidal anti-inflammatory drug.

Aleve Brand name for generic drug anaprox, a nonsteroidal anti-inflammatory drug.

Allodynia Pain from a stimulus that does not ordinarily cause pain.

Alternative medicine Medicine that is out of the mainstream and not always accepted by all conventional medical practitioners.

Amitriptyline Generic name for brand-name drug Elavil, an antidepressant.

Amygdala A part of the brain involved in sexual response, anger, aggression, and fear.

Analgesics Drugs specifically formulated to relieve pain. They include opioids, nonopioids, and combination drugs that have both opioid and nonopioid ingredients.

Anaprox Generic name for brand-name drug Aleve.

Antagonist A substance that neutralizes or counteracts the effects of a drug.

Atarax Brand name for generic drug hydroxyzine, an antihistamine.

Autonomic nervous system Part of the nervous system that helps the body to adapt to changes in the environment; determines how the body responds to stress; regulates the electrical activity of the heart and the movement of the stomach, intestines, and salivary glands; and controls sexual functions and the secretion of insulin.

B

Badofen Brand name for generic drug lioresal, a muscle relaxant.

Basal ganglia An area of the brain responsible for repetitive behaviors, reward experiences, and focusing of attention.

Bentyl Brand name for generic drug dicyclomine, a stomach relaxant.

Body scan Meditative practice that involves lying down and moving the mind through different regions of the body much like a CT scan machine might. Adapted from an ancient Burmese practice.

C

Catapres Brand name for generic drug clonidine, used for high blood pressure and withdrawal from opioids.

Central pain A condition where the brain and nervous system are altered, resulting in feeling more pain.

Cerebellum Structure in the brain that regulates involuntary activities such as breathing, heartbeat, temperature control, and fluid balance; also coordinates movement.

Cerebral cortex A thin layer of tissue in the brain that coats the surface of the cerebrum and cerebellum. Most of the information processing in the brain takes place here.

Cerebrum The largest part of the human brain, associated with higher brain function such as thought and action. It is divided into four sections: the frontal lobe, parietal lobe, occipital lobe, and temporal lobe.

Chi An invisible but very powerful, subtle energy that permeates all things, including the human body.

Chronic pain syndrome (CPS) Pain that has lasted more than six months, may include sleep difficulties, depression, worry, anger, poor memory, inability to concentrate, decreased self-esteem, and a host of other issues and concerns.

Cingulate gyrus A part of the brain that provides a path from the thalamus to the hippocampus and is responsible for the brain's alert system, for focusing attention on emotionally significant events, and for associating memories to smells and pain.

Clonidine Generic name for brand-name drug Catapres, used for high blood pressure and withdrawal from opioids.

Complementary and alternative medicine (CAM) Medical and health care systems, practices, and products not presently considered to be part of conventional medicine. Many complementary medical therapies are used in conjunction with conventional medicine to complement its effects.

Complex regional pain syndrome Chronic pain condition believed to be the result of dysfunction in the central or peripheral nervous system. Generally caused by tissue injury, the symptoms may include changes in color and temperature of the skin over the affected area, with severe burning pain, skin sensitivity, and swelling. In some cases this pain can be incapacitating.

Cymbalta Brand name for generic drug duloxetine, an antidepressant that also decreases neuropathic pain.

CT scan Computerized axial tomography scan, commonly known as a CT or CAT scan; an x-ray procedure that combines numerous x-ray images from a computer to create cross-sectional views of internal organs and structures within the body.

D

Depakote Brand name for generic drug valproic acid, an anticonvulsant medication also used for pain control and bipolar disorder.

Desyrel Brand name for generic drug trazadone, an antidepressant.

Dicyclomine Generic name for brand-name drug Bentyl, a stomach relaxant.

Dopamine A neurotransmitter involved with addiction, love, and the basic reward drives for pleasure; also involved with voluntary movement.

Doshas In Ayurveda, three qualities (vata, pitta, and kapha) that form important characteristics of the body and control the body's activities.

Duloxetine Generic name for brand-name drug Cymbalta, an antidepressant that also decreases neuropathic pain.

Dysphoria A feeling of low energy and irritability, with depressed mood.

E

Effexor Brand name for generic drug venlafexine, an antidepressant.

Elavil Brand name for generic drug amitriptyline, an antidepressant.

Electromyography (EMG) A test that checks the health of the muscles and the nerves that control the muscles.

Endocrine system A collection of glands and organs that produce and regulate hormones that control various functions in the body. It is responsible for many of the body's functions, including metabolism, growth, and sexual development.

Enkephalins One of the three major families of opioid peptides. Enkephalins are amino acids found in the central and peripheral nervous systems and in the inner portion of the adrenal gland, which helps to dull or block pain.

Epinephrine (adrenaline) Increases heart rate, contracts blood vessels, dilates air passages; also involved with the fight-or-flight response governed by the sympathetic nervous system.

F

Fibromyalgia Disorder with primary symptoms of widespread musculoskeletal and soft-tissue pain, severe fatigue, and disturbed sleep. Symptoms may also include muscle twitches and burning sensations. More women than men seem to be afflicted with this condition.

Forebrain The largest and most highly developed part of the brain, consisting of the cerebrum and the structures beneath.

Frontal cortex A thin layer of tissue in the brain that coats the surface of the cerebrum and cerebellum. Most of the information processing in the brain takes place here.

Frontal lobe Area of the brain that controls emotions and development of personality. It is involved with problem solving, memory, language, motor function, impulse control, and social behavior.

Functional magnetic resonance imaging (fMRI) Use of a medical imaging device to map brain activity during specific tasks or sensory processes, including experiencing of pain.

G

Gabapentin Generic name for brand-name drug Neurontin, an anticonvulsant drug also used for pain and mood stabilization.

GABA (gamma-aminobutyric acid) A neurotransmitter that turns off motor neurons, resulting in relaxation and sleepiness.

Graston device Metal instrument that is shaped and contoured to work on and massage specific body parts. It is commonly used in physical therapy to treat soft-tissue injuries to the back, neck, and knee as well as scar tissue from previous surgery.

H

Herpes zoster Virus similar to chicken pox that causes neuropathic pain.

Hindbrain The part of the brain that controls the body's involuntary functions and includes the upper part of the spinal cord, the brain stem, and the cerebellum.

Hippocampus A part of the brain involved in turning short-term memories into long-term memories.

Homeostasis The maintenance of a constant environment within cellular structures. This equilibrium is necessary for cells to stay healthy and fight disease.

Hyperalgesia Exaggerated or distorted pain from a painful stimulus.

Hypothalamus A part of the brain associated with homeostasis, body temperature, pulse, blood pressure, aggression, breathing, and hunger. It is involved in arousal connected with emotional situations, thirst, pleasure, anger, sexual satisfaction, and more, including pain response.

Hypoxia A reduction or shortage of oxygen in the blood.

I

Ibuprofen Generic name for brand-name drug Advil or Motrin.

Individualized drug counseling Therapeutic counseling that focuses directly on reducing or stopping the patient's drug use.

Interoceptive system Highly specialized areas of the brain that mediate motivation to correct internal states and maintain a state of well-being.

Insula Located within the cerebral cortex and associated with body movement, emotional awareness, time perception, perceptual decision making, and a variety of other functions.

J

Johari Window Created by Joseph Luft and Harrington Ingram—hence "Johari"—to help promote self-awareness of personal or group information such as feelings, experiences, views, skills, and so forth, from four perspectives. It is a useful tool for comparing self-perception to public perception and is used as a guide map for developmental improvements.

L

Limbic system A part of the brain linked to olfactory sensation, learning, memory, processing of cognitive data, sexual function, and emotions.

Lioresal Generic name for brand-name drug Baclofen, a muscle relaxant.

M

Matrix Model The therapist acts as both teacher and coach. Interaction between the therapist and the individual seeking treatment is realistic and direct, but not confrontational or parental.

Mechanoreceptive nociceptors Specialized nerves that react to pressure.

Medication-assisted treatment (maintenance) The use of medications, in combination with counseling and behavioral therapies to treat substance use disorders.

Methocarbomal Generic name for brand-name drug Robaxin, a muscle relaxant.

Midbrain The uppermost part of the brain stem that controls some reflex actions, eye movements, other voluntary movements, and many emotions we feel.

Motivational enhancement therapy A client-centered approach to help those with addiction resolve ambivalence about engaging in treatment and stopping drug use.

Motrin Brand name for generic drug ibuprofen, a nonsteroidal anti-inflammatory drug.

MRI Magnetic resonance imaging, commonly known as an MRI scan, a radiology procedure that uses magnetic energy radio waves and a computer to produce images of body structures. The scanner is a tube surrounded by a huge circular magnet, which creates a strong magnetic field as it passes over the patient. Some procedures require a contrast agent that is usually injected into the patient in order to increase the image's accuracy.

Myelin Insulation that protects and insulates neurons. It also aids in the quick transmission of electrical currents carrying information from one nerve cell to the next.

Myofascial Relating to the band of fibrous connective tissue surrounding or holding together muscles, organs, and other soft structures of the body.

N

Naprosyn Brand name for generic drug naproxen, a nonsteroidal anti-inflammatory drug.

Neuromodulators Neurotransmitters involved with sensory transmission, especially pain.

Neurons Also called nerve cells, neurons are excitable cells located in the nervous system that process and transmit information. They are the core of the brain and spinal cord.

Neurontin Brand name for generic drug gabapentin, an anticonvulsant drug also used for pain and mood stabilization.

Neuropathic pain Pain resulting when the nerve fibers or the circuits between the nerves and the brain may have been damaged or injured.

Neuropathy A degenerative disease or disorder of the nervous system.

Neuroplasticity The brain's ability to change and adapt in response to injury or trauma.

Neurotransmitters Chemicals in the brain that transmit nerve impulses across a synapse.

Nociceptors Sensory receptors in the body that send messages to the brain involving painful stimulus.

Norepinephrine A neurotransmitter involved with wakefulness, anxiety, alertness, blood pressure, tone of the blood vessels, and bronchi (air tubes in the lungs).

Nortriptyline Generic name for brand-name drug Pamelor, a sedating antidepressant.

NSAID Nonsteroidal anti-inflammatory drug.

Nucleus accumbens A part of the brain that plays a role in sexual arousal and the "high" from many drugs.

O

Obsessive-compulsive disorder (OCD) An anxiety disorder characterized by recurrent, unwanted thoughts (obsessions) and/or repetitive behaviors (compulsions).

Opioid A chemical substance used to relieve pain through a morphine-like action in the body. The natural class of these drugs is made from the opium poppy. Opioids can be natural, semi-synthetic, or fully synthetic. In this book, "opioids" and "opiates" are used interchangeably, although opioids generally refers to the natural opium alkaloids and the semisynthetics made from them.

Opioid-induced hyperalgesia Condition manifested by an increased or exaggerated response to painful stimuli that occurs in some people who take large doses of opioids to treat chronic pain.

Oxytocin Hormone produced by the pituitary gland that stimulates contraction of the smooth muscle of the uterus.

P

Pamelor Brand name for generic drug nortriptyline, a sedating antidepressant.

Parasympathetic nervous system The "rest and digest" part of the autonomic nervous system, responsible for anxiety reduction, slowing of heart rate, activity of intestines and glands, and relaxing of sphincter muscles.

Physical dependence A condition in which a person's body has adapted to a drug.

Placebo effect Occurs when a person improves or gets better simply by thinking that a treatment or medication is going to help him or her improve or get better.

Plasticity (neuroplasticity) Ability of the brain to reorganize itself by allowing nerve cells to compensate for disease and/or injury and to adjust to changes or new circumstances in the nerve cell's environment.

Polymodal nociceptors Specialized nerves that react to pressure and temperature.

Postherpetic neuralgia Neuropathic pain that occurs after a case caused by the herpes virus.

Prefrontal cortex An area of the brain responsible for planning for the future and taking action. It is also responsible for dopamine pathways and plays a role in addiction and pleasure.

Primal Reflex Release Technique (PRRT) Based on a concept developed by John Jams, PT that believes reflexes can become dysfunctional and create a persistent state of pain. A palpation exam is used to identify areas being held in a tense state. The therapist uses several methods to help the client "release" the tensed areas such as rapid muscle contractions, sustained positioning, and quick tapping.

Prolotherapy A natural technique that stimulates the body to repair painful areas such as tendons and ligaments. It involves the injection of a mildly irritant solution that causes an inflammatory response, stimulating the growth of new ligament and tendon tissue.

Protracted withdrawal A set of signs and symptoms that persist beyond an expected time for acute withdrawal from a substance—alcohol or other drugs. Symptoms may include depression, anxiety, sleep difficulties, and cognitive deficits.

R

Rational recovery (RR) A self-help therapy based on the assumption that psychological difficulties, including addiction, are caused by irrational beliefs that can be understood and overcome through rational self-examination.

Rebound pain Pain that returns even more intensely as a pain-relieving drug wears off.

Referred pain Pain that is felt at a place different from the where the injured or diseased part of the body is located.

Reflex sympathetic dystrophy/causalgia Condition in which symptoms usually include burning pain along the course of a peripheral nerve, tenderness, and soft-tissue swelling out of proportion to the injury.

Relapse The return of symptoms of a disease after a patient has experienced a period of no symptoms/remission. Also refers to a person in recovery who starts to use alcohol or other drugs, gamble, overeat, and so on, after having a period of abstinence.

Relational frame theory A psychological theory of language that focuses on how humans learn language through interactions with the environment. It emphasizes the importance of predicting and influencing events by focusing on manipulating variables in their context.

Robaxin Brand name for generic drug methocarbomal, a muscle relaxant.

S

Secondary gain Usually an unconscious psychological process that allows a person to unwittingly benefit from an undesirable condition by eliciting sympathy or avoiding certain responsibilities.

Self-management and recovery training (SMART) A secular and science-based recovery method using nonconfrontational, motivational, behavioral, and cognitive forms of therapy. Addiction is viewed as a dysfunctional habit rather than a disease.

Sensitization The process by which the nervous system warps and/or magnifies a painful stimulus.

Septum A partition separating two cavities or spaces in the brain that is responsible for modulating impulses between the brain stem and hippocampus.

Serotonin A neurotransmitter involved with memory, emotions, mood, appetite, wakefulness, sleep, and temperature regulation.

Somatosensory cortex Processes input from the various systems in the body that are sensitive to touch. There are a number of different sensory experiences involved in touch.

Substance P A chemical associated with the regulation of mood disorders, anxiety, stress, respiratory rhythm, neurotoxicity, nausea, vomiting, and pain.

Supportive-expressive psychotherapy A time-limited, focused psychotherapy with supportive techniques to help patients feel comfortable in discussing their personal experiences and expressive techniques to help patients identify and work through interpersonal relationship issues.

Sympathetic nervous system The "fight-or-flight" part of the autonomic nervous system, responsible for producing excitation, accelerating the heart rate, constricting blood vessels, dilating the pupils, and raising blood pressure.

T

TENS (transcutaneous electrical nerve stimulation) Small, battery-powered device that produces a vibration or signal intended to interrupt pain transmissions from nerves before they reach the brain.

Thalamus Part of the brain that processes pain.

Thermoreceptive nociceptors Specialized nerves that react to temperature.

Tolerance Requiring more of a medication or substance after an extended period of taking it in order for it to have the same effect as it did when the patient first started taking it.

Trazadone Generic name for the brand-name drug Desyrel, an antidepressant.

Treatment expectancy Influence of a person's beliefs about how well a treatment will work before it is started on how well the treatment actually works—the stronger the expectancy, the better the outcome.

Trigeminal neuralgia Searing, lightning-like pain that shoots through the face. It tends to affect women more often than men, and usually those older than fifty. Attacks can occur spontaneously or result from mild facial stimulation.

V

Valproic acid Generic name for brand-name drug Depakote, an anticonvulsant medication also used for pain control and bipolar disorder.

Values-consistent behavior Behavior that is based on what an individual finds important; actions that are congruent with an individual's values.

Venlafexine Generic name for brand-name drug Effexor, an antidepressant.

Ventral tegmental area An area of the midbrain stem consisting of dopamine pathways; responsible for pleasure.

Vistaril Brand name for generic drug hydroxyzine, an antihistamine.

W

Withdrawal Uncomfortable sensations experienced after abruptly stopping or decreasing the dose of a drug one is dependent on.

Withdrawal-mediated pain Pain that occurs because medication levels are decreasing.

REFERENCES

CHAPTER ONE
What Is Pain?

Bogduk, N., and Merskey, H., editors. *Classification of Chronic Pain: Descriptions of Chronic Pain Syndromes and Definitions of Pain Terms.* 2nd edition. Seattle: IASP Press, 2004.

Brand, P., and Yancey, P. *Pain: The Gift Nobody Wants.* HarperCollins Publishers, 1997.

Colameco, S. *12 Steps for Those Afflicted with Chronic Pain: A Guide to Recovery from Emotional and Spiritual Suffering.* BookSurge, 2005.

Falk, K. M., and Shank, S. L. *Pain Management.* National Center of Continuing Education, Inc., 2005.

National Institute of Neurological Disorders and Stroke. "Pain: Hope through research." December 2001. http://www.ninds.nih.gov/disorders/chronic_pain/detail_chronic_pain.htm.

Peter D. Hart Research Associates. "Americans talk about pain: A survey among adults nationwide conducted for Research!America." August 2003. http://www.researchamerica.org/uploads/poll2003pain.pdf.

Research!America. "Investment in research saves lives and money." Fact Sheet #10. http://www.researchamerica.org/uploads/factsheet10pain.pdf.

Trescot, A. M., Boswell, M. V., Atluri, S. L., et al. "Opioid guidelines." *Pain Physician* 9, no. 1 (2006): 4–6.

CHAPTER TWO
Chronic Pain Never Goes Away

AboutKidsHealth. "Factors affecting pain assessment." The Hospital for Sick Children. 2005. http://www.aboutkidshealth.ca/En/ResourceCentres/Pain/PainAssessment/FactorsAffectingPainAssessment/Pages/default.aspx.

American Pain Foundation. "Pain facts & figures." 2006. http://www. painfoundation.org/media/resources/pain-facts-figures.html.

Bair, M. J., Robinson, R. L., Eckert, G. J., Stang, et al. "Impact of pain on depression treatment response in primary care." *Psychosomatic Medicine* 66 (2004): 17–22.

Centers for Disease Control and Prevention. U.S. Department of Health and Human Services. NCHS Data Brief, No. 30, March 2010. "Prevalence and management of pain, by race and dementia among nursing home residents: United States, 2004." http://www.cdc.gov/nchs/data/databriefs/db30.pdf

Farber, P. L., Blustein, J., Gordon, E., and Neveloff, N. "Pain: Ethics, culture, and informed consent to relief." *Journal of Law, Medicine & Ethics* 24, no. 4 (1996): 348–359.

Holdcroft, A., and Power, I. "Recent developments: Management of pain." *British Medical Journal* 326 (2003): 635–639.

International Association for the Study of Pain. "Pain and ethnicity." *Pain Clinical Updates* IX, no. 4, 2001.

Linton, S. J. *Understanding Pain for Better Clinical Practice: A Psychological Perspective.* Elsevier, 2005.

Mayo Clinic. "How you feel pain." Mayo Foundation for Medical Education and Research. 2007.

Medical Disability Advisor. "Medical Disability Guidelines: Pain, Chronic." http://www.mdguidelines.com/pain-chronic.

National Center for Health Statistics. *Health, United States, 2006,* with chart book on trends in the health of Americans with special feature on pain. CDC National Center for Health Statistics Press, 2006.

National Institute of Neurological Disorders and Stroke. "Study suggests improved treatments for neuropathic pain." National Institutes of Health http:// www.ninds.nih.gov/news_and_events/news_articles/news_article_pain_MMPs. htm.

National Institute of Neurological Disorders and Stroke. "Pain: Hope through research." April 2011. http://www.ninds.nih.gov/disorders/chronic_pain/detail_ chronic_pain.htm.

National Pain Foundation. "Pain and depression." http://nationalpainfoundation. org/articles/98/pain-and-depression.

Senden, I. P. M., Wetering, M. D., Eskes, T. K., et al. "Labor pain: A comparison of parturients in a Dutch and an American teaching hospital." *Obstetrics & Gynecology* 71 (1988): 541–544.

Society for Neuroscience. "Gender and pain." *Brain Briefings*, May 2007. http:// web.sfn.org/index.aspx?pagename=brainBriefings_Gender_and_Pain.

World Health Organization. "Cancer." Fact Sheet No. 297. February 2011. http:// www.who.int/mediacentre/factsheets/fs297/en/index.html.

Zinke, J. "Culture, pain, and pain research." *American Pain Society Bulletin* 17, no. 2 (2007). http://ampainsoc.org/pub/bulletin/sum07/research1.htm.

CHAPTER THREE
No Brain, No Pain

Baliki, M. N., Geha, P. Y., Apkarian, A. V., and Chialvo, D. R. "Beyond feeling: Chronic pain hurts the brain, disrupting the default-mode network dynamics." *The Journal of Neuroscience* 28, no. 6 (2008): 1398–1403.

Begley, S. "The lotus and the synapse." *Newsweek*, March 25, 2008. http://www. newsweek.com/blogs/lab-notes/2008/03/25/the-lotus-and-the-synapse.html.

Carmichael, M. "The changing science of pain." *Newsweek*, June 4, 2007.

Choi, J. T., and Bastian, A. J. "Adaptation reveals independent control networks for human walking." *Nature Neuroscience* 10 (2007): 1055–1062.

Craig, A. D. "How do you feel? Interoception: The sense of the physiological condition of the body." *Current Opinion in Neurobiology* August 2003 13(4): 500–505.

Craig, A. D. "Interoception: The sense of the physiological condition of the body." *Neurobiology* 4 (August 13, 2003): 500–505.

Flor, H. "Pain, learning and brain plasticity: Implications for treatment." Department of Clinical and Cognitive Neuroscience, University of Heidelberg, Mannheim, Germany.

Mackey, S. "The strain in pain lies mainly in the brain." Stanford School of Medicine, Pain Management Center. http://snap1.stanford.edu/research.

National Institutes of Health. *The Brain: Our Sense of Self.* Colorado Springs: BSCS, 2005. http://science.education.nih.gov/supplements/nih4/self/guide/ nih_self_curr-supp.pdf.

Ohayon, M. M., and Schatzberg, A.F. "Using chronic pain to predict depressive morbidity in the general population. *Arch Gen Psychiatry* 60, no. 1 (2003): 39–47.

Richeimer, S. "Understanding neuropathic pain." USC Pain Management. http://spineuniverse.com/displayarticle.php/article1614.html.

Rodriguez-Gil, G. "The plastic brain." California Deaf-Blind Services, 2005.

Wager, T. D., Rilling, J. K., Smith, E. E., et al. "Placebo-induced changes in fMRI in the anticipation and experience of pain." *Science* 303, no. 5661 (2004): 1162–1167.

CHAPTER FOUR
Falling Down the Rabbit Hole
Opioids and Chronic Pain

Ballantyne, J., and Mao, J. "Long-term opioid use in some is associated with abnormal sensitivity to pain." *The New England Journal of Medicine* 349, no. 20 (November 13, 2003): 1943–1953.

Bass, F. "Pain medicine use has nearly doubled." The Associated Press, August 20, 2007.

Centers for Disease Control and Prevention. "Unintentional drug poisoning in the United States." July 2010. http://www.cdc.gov/homeandrecreationalsafety/ poisoning/brief.htm.

Duensing, L. "Prescribing opioids: The changing landscape." *The Pain Practitioner* 15, no. 2 (2005): 24–31.

Gourlay, D. L., Heit, H. A., and Almahrezi, A. "Universal precautions in pain medicine: A rational approach to the treatment of chronic pain. *Pain Medicine* 6, no. 2 (March/April 2005): 107–112.

International Association for the Study of Pain. "Reducing the risk of opioid misuse in persistent pain: Commentary on Jamison et al." *Pain* 150 (2010).

Leavitt, S. B. "Iatrogenic opioid-use problems: What's the risk?" *Pain Treatment Topics e-Briefing* 2, no. 1 (2007). http://pain-topics.org/pdf/e-Briefing-Vol2-No1-2007.pdf.

National Institutes of Health. "Prescription pain medicines—An addictive path?" Fall 2007. http://www.nlm.nih.gov/medlineplus/magazine/issues/fall07/articles/fall07pg22a.html.

National Institute of Neurological Disorders and Stroke. "Brain basics: Know your brain." 2007. http://www.ninds.nih.gov/disorders/brain_basics/know_your_brain.htm.

National Institute on Drug Abuse. "Prescription and over-the-counter medications." National Institutes of Health. June 2009. http://www.nida.nih.gov/infofacts/painmed.html.

Ohayon, M. M., and Schatzberg, A. F. "Using chronic pain to predict depressive morbidity in the general population." *Arch Gen Psychiatry* 60, no. 1 (January 2003): 39–47.

Roy, S., and Loh, H. H. "Effects of opioids on the immune system." *Neurochemical Research* 21, no. 11 (1996): 1375–1386.

Savage, S., Covington, E. C., Gilson, A. M., et al. "Public policy statement on the rights and responsibilities of healthcare professionals in the use of opioids for the treatment of pain." American Academy of Pain Medicine, American Pain Society, and American Society of Addiction Medicine, 2004.

Strassels, S. A. "Economic burden of prescription opioid misuse and abuse." *Journal of Managed Care Pharmacy* 15, no. 7 (2009): 556–562.

White, J. M. "Pleasure into pain: The consequences of long-term opioid use." *Addictive Behaviors* 29 (2004): 1311–1324.

World Health Organization. "WHO normative guidelines on pain management." Geneva, 2007. http://www.who.int/medicines/areas/quality_safety/delphi_study_pain_guidelines.pdf.

CHAPTER FIVE
Drug Addiction

American Psychiatric Association. *Diagnostic and Statistical Manual of Mental Disorders DSM-IV,* fourth edition. American Psychiatric Association, 1994.

Baliki, M. N., Geha, P. Y., Apkarian, V. A., and Chialvo, D. R. "Beyond feeling: Chronic pain hurts the brain, disrupting the default-mode network dynamics." *The Journal of Neuroscience* 28, no. 6 (2008): 1398–1403.

Berger, A. M., Portenoy, R. K., and Weissman, D. E. *Principles and Practice of Palliative Care and Supportive Oncology*. Lippincott Williams & Wilkins, 2002.

Centers for Disease Control and Prevention, U.S. Department of Health and Human Services. Morbidity and Mortality Weekly Report, Supplement, Vol. 60. "CDC health disparities and inequalities report—United States, 2011." http://www.cdc.gov/mmwr/pdf/other/su6001.pdf.

Craig, A. D. "Interoception: The sense of the physiological condition of the body." *Neurobiology* 4 (August 13, 2003): 500–505.

Craig, A. D.. "How do you feel? Interoception: The sense of the physiological condition of the body." *Neuroscience* 3, no. 8 (August 2002): Review 655–666.

Drug Abuse Warning Network. "Area profiles of drug-related mortality." DAWN Series D-27, DHHS Publication No. (SMA) 05-4023, Rockville, MD, March 2005.

Hanson, R. *Self-Management of Chronic Pain: Patient Handbook*. Long Beach: VA Healthcare System. http://www.arachnoiditis.info/website_captures/chronicpainhandbook/Mental%20Health-%20VA%20Long%20Beach%20Healthcare%20System.htm

International Association for the Study of Pain. "Acceptance of chronic pain: Component analysis and a revised assessment method." *Pain* 107 (2004).

Lemonick, M. D. "How we get addicted." *Time*, 2007. http://www.time.com/time/magazine/article/0,9171,1640436,00.html.

Leshner, A. I. "Addiction is a brain disease." *Issues in Science & Technology* 17, no. 3 (March 22, 2001). http://www.issues.org/17.3/leshner.htm.

National Association for Children of Alcoholics. "Children of addicted parents: Important facts." http://www.nacoa.net/pdfs/addicted.pdf.

National Council for Community Behavioral Healthcare. "Preventing and treating substance use disorders: A comprehensive approach." http://www.thenationalcouncil.org/galleries/policy-file/Substance%20Use%20Disorders.pdf.

National Institute on Drug Abuse. "Drugged driving." National Institutes of Health. http://www.nida.nih.gov/PDF/Infofacts/driving.pdf.

National Institute on Drug Abuse. "Drugs, brains and behavior—the science of addiction." National Institutes of Health. http://drugabuse.gov/scienceofaddiction/sciofaddiction.pdf.

National Institute on Drug Abuse. "NIDA-supported researchers use brain imaging to deepen understanding of addiction." *NIDA Notes Special Report: Brain Imaging Research* 11, no. 5 (November/December 1996). http://www.drugabuse.gov/NIDA_Notes/NNVol11N5/Deepen.html.

National Institute on Drug Abuse. NIDA for Teens. "Facts on drugs: HIV, AIDS, and drug abuse." National Institutes of Health. http://teens.drugabuse.gov/facts/facts_hiv1.php.

National Institute on Drug Abuse. Topics in Brief. "Prescription drug abuse May 2011." National Institutes of Health. http://www.nida.nih.gov/pdf/tib/prescription.pdf.

Nugent, F. S., Penick, E. C., and Kauer, J. A. "Opioids block long-term potentiation of inhibitory synapses." *Nature* 446 (2007): 1086–1090.

Passik, S. D. "Aberrant drug-taking behaviors in pain patients." PowerPoint presentation at the meeting of the U.S. Food and Drug Administration. 2003. Anesthetic and Life Support Drugs Advisory Committee, Bethesda, Maryland.

Portenoy, R. K. "Opioid therapy for chronic nonmalignant pain: Clinician's perspective." *Journal of Law, Medicine and Ethics* 24, no. 4 (1996): 296–309.

Rosenburg, T. "When is a pain doctor a drug pusher?" *The New York Times*, June 17, 2007, cover story.

Schneider, J. "Addiction and chronic pain." The National Pain Foundation. http://www.nationalpainfoundation.org/articles/134/addiction-and-chronic-pain.

Substance Abuse and Mental Health Services Administration. *Results from the 2006 National Survey on Drug Use and Health: National Findings.* 2007. Rockville, MD: Office of Applied Studies, NSDUH Series H-32, DHHS Publication No. SMA 07-4293.

Substance Abuse and Mental Health Services Administration, Office of Applied Studies. *Results from the 2009 National Survey on Drug Use and Health: National Findings.* 2010.

Substance Abuse and Mental Health Services Administration, Office of Applied Studies. "The DAWN Report: Trends in emergency department visits involving nonmedical use of narcotic pain relievers." Rockville, Maryland, June 2010.

Substance Abuse and Mental Health Services Administration, Office of Applied Studies. . "The New DAWN Report: Emergency department visits involving nonmedical use of selected pharmaceuticals." Issue 23, 2006.

The National Center on Addiction and Substance Abuse at Columbia University. "Shoveling up II: The impact of substance abuse on federal, state and local budgets." May 2009. http://www.casacolumbia.org/articlefiles/380-ShovelingUpII.pdf.

World Health Organization. *International Statistical Classification of Diseases and Related Health Problems, 10th Revision.* WHO/DIMDI, 2007. http://www.who.int/classifications/apps/icd/icd10online.

CHAPTER SIX
"I Just Don't *Feel* Good . . ."
Emotions and Suffering

Cobb, L. A., Thomas, G. I., Dillard, D. H., et al. "An evaluation of internal mammary artery ligation by a double-blind technique." *New England Journal of Medicine* 2650 (1959): 1115–18.

Colameco, S. *12 Steps for Those Afflicted with Chronic Pain: A Guide to Recovery from Emotional and Spiritual Suffering.* BookSurge, 2005.

Moffitt, P. "Awakening in the body." *Shambhala Sun,* September 2007.

Price, D. "Multisensory integration in pain and consciousness." *The Journal of Pain* 8, no. 3 (1999).

Scientific Blogging. "Nucleus accumbens and the placebo effect." http://www.science20.com/news/nucleus_accumbens_and_the_placebo_effect.

Siegel, R. D., Urdang, M. H., and Johnson, D. R. *Back Sense: A Revolutionary Approach to Halting the Cycle of Chronic Back Pain.* New York: Broadway Books, 2002.

Stewart-Patterson, C. "Working with chronic pain." *Shambhala Sun,* May 2003.

Vogt, B. A. "Pain and emotion interactions in subregions of the cingulated gyrus." *Nature Reviews Neuroscience* 6 (July 2005): 533–544.

Wade, J. B., Price, D. D., Hamer, R. M., et al. "An emotional component analysis of chronic pain." *Pain* 40, no. 3 (1990): 303–310.

Wray, N. "Arthroscopic knee surgery no better than placebo surgery." *New England Journal of Medicine* 347, no. 2 (2002): 81–88, 132–133.

CHAPTER SEVEN
Working with Thoughts and Emotions

Chödrön, P. *Comfortable with Uncertainty*. Shambhala Publications, 2002.

deCharms, R. C., Maeda, F., Glover, G. H., et al. "Control over brain activation and pain learned by using real-time functional MRI." *PNAS* 102, no. 51: 18626–18631.

Hanson, R. *Self-Management of Chronic Pain: Patient Handbook*. Long Beach: VA Healthcare System. http://www.arachnoiditis.info/website_captures/chronicpainhandbook/Mental%20Health-%20VA%20Long%20Beach%20Healthcare%20System.htm.

National Association of Cognitive-Behavioral Therapists. "What is cognitive-behavioral therapy?" 1996–2008. http://nacbt.org/whatiscbt.htm.

CHAPTER EIGHT
What Is Pain Recovery?
A Solution to Your Suffering from Chronic Pain

McCracken, L. M., and Vowles, K. E. "Psychological flexibility and traditional pain management strategies in relation to patient functioning with chronic pain: An examination of a revised instrument." *Journal of Pain* 8, no. 9 (2007): 700–707.

McCracken, L. M., and Zhao-O'Brien, J. "General psychological acceptance and chronic pain: There is more to accept than the pain itself." *European Journal of Pain*, no. 14 (2010): 170–175.

Pohl, M., Szabo, F., Jr., Shiode, D., and Hunter, R. *Pain Recovery: How to Find Balance and Reduce Suffering from Chronic Pain*. Central Recovery Press, 2009.

Vowles, K. E., and McCracken, L. M. "Acceptance and values-based action in chronic pain: A study of treatment effectiveness and process." *Journal of Clinical Counseling and Psychology* 76, no. 3 (2008): 397–407.

Vowles, K. E., McCracken, L. M., and Eccleston, C. "Patient functioning and catastrophizing in chronic pain: The mediating effects of acceptance." *Health Psychology* 27, no. 2 (supp.) (2008): S136–S143.

CHAPTER NINE
Families Hurt Too

Bufalari, L., Aprile, T., Avenanti, A., et al. "Empathy for pain and touch in the human somatosensory cortex." *Cerebral Cortex* 17, no. 11 (2007): 2553–2561.

Doherty, W. J., and Baird, M. A. *Family Therapy and Family Medicine: Toward the Primary Care of Families*. New York: The Guilford Press, 1983.

Hanson, R. *Self-Management of Chronic Pain: Patient Handbook*. Long Beach: VA Healthcare System. http://www.arachnoiditis.info/website_captures/chronicpainhandbook/Mental%20Health-%20VA%20Long%20Beach%20Healthcare%20System.htm.

Jackson, P. L., Meltzoff, A., and Decety, J. "How do we perceive the pain of others? A window into the neural processes involved in empathy." *Neuroimage* 24, no. 3 (2005): 771–779.

Saarela, M. V., Hlushchuck, Y., de C. Williams, et al. "The compassionate brain: Humans detect intensity of pain from another's face." *Cerebral Cortex (Oxford)* 17, no. 1 (2007): 230–237.

Silver, J. *Chronic Pain and the Family, A New Guide*. Harvard University Press, 2004.

Singer, T., Seymour, B., O'Doherty, J., Kaube, et al. "Empathy for pain involves the affective but not sensory components of pain." *Science* 20, no. 5661 (February 2004): 1157–1162.

Society for Neuroscience. "Findings on pain, including how a spouse can spur the sense, provide new insights." 2002. http://www.sfn.org/index.cfm?pagename=news_11032002a.

von Bertalanffy, L. *General Systems Theory*. George Braziller, 1976.

CHAPTER TEN
Treatment Modalities

American Cancer Society. "Cancer facts & figures." 2010. http://www.cancer.org/acs/groups/content/@epidemiologysurveilance/documents/document/acspc-026238.pdf.

American Cancer Society. "Find support and treatment, turmeric." 2008. http://www.cancer.org/Treatment/TreatmentsandSideEffects/ ComplementaryandAlternativeMedicine/HerbsVitaminsandMinerals/ turmeric?sitearea=ETO.

American Music Therapy Association. "Music therapy and Music-Based Interventions in the Treatment and Management of Pain: Selected References and Findings." 2010. http://www.musictherapy.org/factsheets/MT%20Pain%20 2010.pdf.

Bassett, C. A., Mitchell, S. N., and Gaston S. R. "Pulsing electromagnetic field treatment in un-united fractures and failed arthrodeses." *Journal of the American Medical Association* 247, no. 5 (1982).

Bronfort, G., Haas, M., Evans, R. L., and Bouter, L. M. "Efficacy of spinal manipulation and mobilization for low back pain and neck pain: A systematic review and best evidence synthesis." *Spine* 4, no. 3 (2004): 335–356.

"Cherries pack anti-gout power." *Prevention* (2004). http://www.prevention. com/health/nutrition/food-remedies/cherries-fight-gout-and-arthritis/article/ d6fb50d1fa803110VgnVCM10000013281eac.

Eye Movement Desensitization and Reprocessing Institute, Inc. http://www.emdr. com/.

http://www.emdrworkshops.com/aboutemdr.htm.

Gagnier, J. J., vanTulder, M., Bermann, B., and Bombardier, C. "Herbal medicine for low back pain." Cochrane Reviews, 2006. http://www.cochrane.org/reviews/ en/ab004504.html.

Galarraga, B., Ho, M., Youssef, H. M., et al. "Cod liver oil (n-3 fatty acids) as a nonsteroidal anti-inflammatory drug sparing agent in rheumatoid arthritis." *Rheumatology* (Oxford) 47, no. 5 (2008): 665–669.

Health. "Four ways yoga relieves low back pain." http://www.health.com/health/ condition-article/print/0,,20189616,00.html.

Kabat-Zinn, J. *Full Catastrophe Living*. New York: Bantam Doubleday Dell Publishing Group, Inc., 1990.

Lindner, C. "Altering the pain experience: Hypnotherapy for pain management." HypnoGenesis. http://www.hypnos.co.uk/hypnomag/lindner.htm.

Marcus, D. A. "Treatment of nonmalignant chronic pain." *American Family Physician.* http://www.aafp.org/afp/20000301/1331.html.

Morley, S., Eccleston, C., and Williams, A. "Systematic review and meta-analysis of randomized controlled trials of cognitive behavior therapy and behavior therapy for chronic pain in adults, excluding headaches." *Pain* 80: 1–13.

Moss, D. "Biofeedback, mind-body medicine, and the higher limits of human nature." Association for Applied Psychophysiology and Biofeedback. http://www.aapb.org/articles_interest_human_nature.html.

National Center for Complementary and Alternative Medicine. National Institutes of Health. "An introduction to chiropractic." http://nccam.nih.gov/health/chiropractic.

National Center for Complimentary and Alternative Medicine. National Institutes of Health. "Magnets for Pain." http://nccam.nih.gov/health/magnet/magnetsforpain.htm.

National Center for Complimentary and Alternative Medicine. National Institutes of Health. "Massage Therapy." http://nccam.nih.gov/health/massage/.

National Center for Complimentary and Alternative Medicine. National Institutes of Health. "Reiki." http://nccam.nih.gov/health/reiki/.

Omoni, A. O., and Aluko, R. E. "Soybean foods and their benefits: Potential mechanisms of action." *Nutrition Reviews* 63, no. 8 (2005): 272–283.

Peck, I. L., and Peck, R. A. "How traditional Chinese medicine views the human body in relation to the disease process." *The Pain Practitioner* 15, no. 1 (2005): 21–26.

Rushton, D. N. "Electrical stimulation in the treatment of pain." *Disability and Rehabilitation* 24, no. 8 (2002): 407–415.

Rusy, L. M. "Acupuncture provides pain relief for many patients." Health Link, Medical College of Wisconsin, 2003–2008. http://www.mcw.edu/clinicalinformatics/healthlink.htm.

StopPain.org. "Pain management, complimentary approaches." http://www.healingchronicpain.org/content/introduction/comp_nutrition.asp.

University of Texas, M. D. Anderson Cancer Center. "Teaching the art of aromatherapy to soothe and heal." ScienceDaily, 2006. http://www.sciencedaily.com/releases/2006/08/060825201430.htm.

U.S. Department of Health and Human Services. "Physical activity fundamental to preventing disease." 2002. http://aspe.hhs.gov/health/reports/physicalactivity/.

Usui, M. "History of Dr. Usui Sensei 1865–1926." http://www.reiki.nu/history/usui/usui.html. Copyright 2000–2004, www.reiki.nu.

Woolston, C. "Massage for pain relief." HealthDay, 2006. http://consumer.healthday.com/encyclopedia/article.asp?AID=645793.

World Chiropractic Alliance. "Consumer education." http://www.worldchiropracticalliance.org/consumer/history.htm.

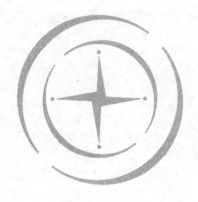

A Day without Pain Blog
adaywithoutpain.com

American Academy of Medical Acupuncture (AAMA)
medicalacupuncture.org
Phone: (323) 937-5514

American Academy of Pain Medicine (AAPM)
painmed.org
Phone: (847) 375-4731

American Chronic Pain Association (ACPA)
theacpa.org
Phone: (800) 533-3231

The American Massage Therapy Association (AMTA)
amtamassage.org
Phone: (877) 905-2700

American Music Therapy Association (AMTA)
musictherapy.org
Phone: (301) 589-3300

American Pain Foundation (APF)
painfoundation.org
Phone: (888) 615-PAIN (7246)

American Pain Society (APS)
ampainsoc.org
Phone: (847) 375-4715

American Physical Therapy Association (APTA)
apta.org
Phone: (800) 999–APTA (2782)

American Psychological Association (APA)
apa.org
Phone: (800) 374-2721

American Society of Addiction Medicine (ASAM)
asain.org
Phone: (301) 656-3920

Andrew Weil, MD
drweil.com

Association for Behavioral and Cognitive Therapies (ABCT)
abct.org
Phone: (212) 647-1890

EMDR International Association
emdna.org
Phone: (866) 451-5200

How to Meditate
how-to-meditate.org

International Association for the Study of Pain (IASP)
iasp-pain.org
Phone: (206) 283-0311

Las Vegas Recovery Center (LVRC)
Lasvegasrecovery.com
Phone: (702) 515-1374

Meditation Society of America
meditationsociety.com

National Association of Cognitive Behavioral Therapists (NACBT)
nacbt.org
Phone: (800) 853-1135

National Association of Holistic Aromatherapy (NAHA)
naha.org
Phone: (509) 325-3419

National Center for Complementary and Alternative Medicine (NCCAM)
National Institutes of Health (NIH)
nccamnih.gov
Phone: (888) 644-6226

National Institute on Drug Abuse (NIDA)
National Institutes of Health (NIH)
nida.nih.gov
Phone: (301) 443-1124

National Institute of Neurological Disorders and Stroke (NINDS)
National Institutes of Health (NIH)
ninds.nih.gov
Phone: (800) 352-9424

National Pain Foundation
nationalpainfoundation.org

Office of National Drug Control Policy (ONDCP)
whitehousedrugpolicy.gov
Phone: (800) 666-3332

Pilates Method Alliance (PMA)
pilatesmethodalliance.org
Phone: (866) 573-4945

Qigong Institute
qigonginstitute.org

Reiki.nu
reiki.nu

Society for Neuroscience
sfn.org
Phone: (202) 962-4000

Stanford School of Medicine Pain Management Center
med.stanford.edu

Substance Abuse and Mental Health Services Administration (SAMHSA)
samhsa.gov
Phone: (877)-SAMHSA-7 (877-726-4727)

World Chiropractic Alliance
worldchiropracticafliance.org
Phone: (800) 347-1011

World Health Organization
who.int
Phone: (+ 41 22) 791 21 11 *(Switzerland)*

Yoga Alliance
yogaafliance.org
Phone: (877) 964-2255

ALSO AVAILABLE FROM CENTRAL RECOVERY PRESS
www.centralrecoverypress.com

PAIN RECOVERY

*Pain Recovery: How to Find Balance and Reduce Suffering
from Chronic Pain*
Mel Pohl, MD, FASAM; Frank J. Szabo, Jr., LADC; Dan Shiode, Ph.D.; Rob
Hunter, Ph.D. • $20.95 US • ISBN-13: 978-0-9799869-9-4

*Pain Recovery for Families: How to Find Balance When Someone Else's
Chronic Pain Becomes Your Problem Too*
Mel Pohl, MD, FASAM; Frank J. Szabo, Jr., LADC; Dan Shiode, Ph.D.; Rob
Hunter, Ph.D. • $20.95 US • ISBN-13: 978-0-9818482-3-5

Meditations for Pain Recovery
Tony Greco • $16.95 US • ISBN 13: 978-0-9818482-8-0

INSPIRATIONAL

The Truth Begins with You: Reflections to Heal Your Spirit
Claudia Black, Ph.D. • $17.95 US • ISBN-13: 978-1-9362-9061-1

*Above and Beyond: 365 Meditations for Transcending Chronic
Pain and Illness*
J.S. Dorian • $15.95 US • ISBN-13: 978-1-9362-9066-6

Guide Me in My Recovery: Prayers for Times of Joy and Times of Trial
Rev. John T. Farrell, Ph.D. • $12.95 US • ISBN-13: 978-1-936290-00-0
Special hardcover gift edition: $19.95 US • ISBN-13: 978-1-936290-02-4

The Soul Workout: Getting and Staying Spiritually Fit
Helen H. Moore • $12.95 US • ISBN-13: 978-0-9799869-8-7

Tails of Recovery: Addicts and the Pets That Love Them
Nancy A. Schenck • $19.95 US • ISBN-13: 978-0-9799869-6-3

Of Character: Building Assets in Recovery
Denise D. Crosson, Ph.D. • $12.95 US • ISBN-13: 978-0-9799869-2-5

MEMOIRS

Leave the Light On: A Memoir of Recovery and Self-Discovery
Jennifer Storm • $14.95 US • ISBN-13: 978-0-9818482-2-8

The Mindful Addict: A Memoir of the Awakening of a Spirit
Tom Catton • $18.95 US • ISBN-13: 978-0-9818482-7-3

Becoming Normal: An Ever-Changing Perspective
Mark Edick • $14.95 US • ISBN-13: 978-0-9818482-1-1

Dopefiend: A Father's Journey from Addiction to Redemption
Tim Elhajj • $16.95 US • ISBN 13: 978-1-936290-63-5